# *Find Your Happetite*

*Eat What You Want and Be
Happy With Your (Perfect) Weight*

*By*

*Sue Zbornik, MSc., APD*

**FIND YOUR HAPPETITE** Copyright 2011 by SUSAN ZBORNIK

All rights reserved. No part of this book may be used or reproduced in any manner whatsoever without written permission from SUSAN ZBORNIK, except as provided by the United States of America copyright law or in the case of brief quotations embodied in articles and reviews.

The scanning, uploading and distribution of this book via the Internet or via any other means without the permission of the publisher is illegal and punishable by law.

Please purchase only authorized electronic editions and do not participate in or encourage electronic piracy of copyrighted materials. Your support of the author's rights is sincerely appreciated.

Book design and layout by Perseus Design

ISBN 978-1-935723-37-0

Printed in the United States of America

First Printing: 2011

The information contained in this book is based on the research and personal and professional experiences of the author. It is not intended as a substitute for consulting with health care professionals. Any attempt to diagnose and treat an illness should be done under the care of a health care professional.

*Dedication*

This book is dedicated to everyone seeking their happetite...

# *Acknowledgements*

Thank you, Thank you, Thank you!

For trusting me and letting me into your lives: my clients past and present. Your courage and strength are amazing (and deepest apologies to anyone I put on a restricted diet early in my career).

For making clinic days fun and interesting: The Meridian Clinic Team at Total Heath Care - Associate Professor Michael Kohn, Vicki Hewson, Felicity Spencer and the other brilliant professional and office staff at Total Health Care.

For teaching me what I could never have learnt on my own: I thank the community of caring and highly evolved people who work here in Australia in the treatment of eating disorders - especially Hazel Williams, Tara MacGregor, Helen Storey, Liz Frig, Alison Wakefield, Nerissa Soh, Susan Hart, Gabriella Heruc, Kylie Richardson and other members of the Dietitian's Association of Australia Eating Disorders Interest Group, past and present. I am also incredibly grateful for my work colleagues over the years at the University of Wisconsin Hospital and Clinics where I first started working in the area of eating disorders (thank you Judy Reinke and Marci Braun); The St. George Hospital, The South Eastern Sydney Area Health Service Community Nutrition Unit, The Royal Prince Alfred Hospital, and Wesley Private Hospital (now the Peter Beumont Eating Disorders Unit).

For inspiration: Ellyn Satter, whose workshop on natural eating in Madison, Wisconsin in 1985 turned my career onto a new path and whose books still inform my work; Judith and Jenny McFadden, a mother and daughter duo from Sydney who furthered my knowledge on appetite-driven eating with NECTAR – Natural Eating, Control Theory and Results; all the authors, researchers and writers whose books and articles fill my shelves and nourish my mind.

For his love and grace, and for helping me to expand my world: my deceased husband Andrew Thompson.

For my family in the USA: My mother Helen Zbornik whose beautiful gardens uplift the soul; my deceased father, Adrian, who tilled the earth of our Iowa farm with love; my sisters Sarah, Cathy and Julie and my brothers John and Steve. Without you my life would have been very dull! For loving my siblings so well: Carol Bouska Zbornik, Dave Magner and Kurt Neyens. And for bringing joy to my life, my beautiful nieces and nephews: Hannah, Stephen James, Benjamin, Samuel, Andrew and Jacob.

For listening to my joys and sorrows and brightening my days and years, I thank my family of friends worldwide, especially: Sarah Magner, Christina Harris, Maryella Hatfield, Joy Moulieri, Anne Cummins, Jean-Marc Maissin, Jen Ward, Tara MacGregor, Carl Bonwick, Sandra Napoli, Mark Phillips, Anna K Phillips, Louise Kanis, Drew Warne-Smith, Mary Kay Aide, Emmanuelle Guenot, Martina Chippendall, Leonice Holthaus, Sara Schnadt, Lori Smetana, Mike Woodson, Dave and Marie Morris, Patrick and Pam Murray, Chris and Sally Thompson.

## Acknowledgements

For opening me to the wonders of the unseen and helping me heal and accept: Lynette Arkadie, Joy Moulieri, Saleema Ladhani, Natali Jocelyn, Ben Hendrickson, Caterina Pellegrino, Alicia Power, Gossamer Cooney, Carol Maher and Jann Jerabek. You each are earth angels of the highest order.

For his brilliance and help when no one else could: Dr. Phillip Van Zanden at the UNSW Health Service. His dedication and persistence has allowed me to learn more about the physiology of my body than all my years of University. Thanks to "Dr Phil", I feel better than ever.

For helping me get this book out of my head and onto the page: my writing coach Ann McIndoo and her team. You are phenomenal! Thanks also to Roland Fishman and Kathleen Allen at The Sydney Writer's Studio for their invaluable help along the way; and to my Australian editor Vanessa Cavasinni.

For reading early drafts and providing suggestions that made this book much better than it would have been: Tara MacGregor, Sarah Magner, Associate Professor Michael Kohn, Jean-Marc Maissin, Wendy McAra, Jen Ward, Albert Ho, Helen Zbornik, Helen Storey and Anne Cummins.

For his strident research and fact-checking: Albert Ho.

For her creativity, friendship and the word "Happetite": Cecilia Persson.

For her beautiful artwork: Jill Ryan; and for their fine graphics skills, Sarah Magner and Sam Glasheen.

For his guidance: my publisher, the wunderkind Justin Sachs, at Motivational Press.

For his boundless love and for getting me out in nature each day: my beautiful pooch Louie.

Lastly, for having the courage to answer the knock of my soul on the door of my life: I thank myself for working through my fears, doubts and insecurities. My soul may have had a plan, but it was very challenging to follow that directive!

# Contents

                                                                                                        *Page*

*The Seven Principles of Happetite* ...................................................... 17

*Principle One: Understanding Your Eating* ......................................... 37
    *Lesson 1 – The Eating Continuum* ................................................. 37
    *Lesson 2 – Self Acceptance* ............................................................. 49
    *Lesson 3 – The Diet-Binge Cycle* .................................................... 54
    *Lesson 4 – Breaking the Diet-Binge Cycle* ..................................... 67

*Principle Two: Understanding Your Happetite* ................................... 73
    *Lesson 5 – DYE-IT (Not Diet) – Ceasing Dieting Behaviours* ....... 74
    *Lesson 6 – How Food Rules Affect Our Decisions* ....................... 82
    *Lesson 7 – Good Food/Bad Food Myths* ....................................... 86
    *Lesson 8 – Have You Ever Been a Normal Eater?* ......................... 97

*Principle Three: Clearing the Physical Challenges* ............................ 109
    *Lesson 9 - Metabolism Basics: Food Intake and Activity* .............. 110
    *Lesson10 – Digestion: Absorption and Malabsorption* ................ 121
    *Lesson 11 – Hormonal Influences* ................................................. 128
    *Lesson 12 – Taking it Further: Food Intolerance* ......................... 139
    *Lesson 13 – Taking it Further: Xenoestrogens* ............................. 141

*Principle Four: Addressing the Emotional Barriers* .......................... 149
    *Lesson 14 – Psychological Effects of Dieting* ................................ 152

Lesson 15 – Acceptance of Weight and Appetite ............................ 155
Lesson 16 – The Potion: Emotion ................................................... 160

*Principle Five: Motivating Yourself for Change* ............................. 171
Lesson 17 – Getting Ready .............................................................. 172
Lesson 18 – The Problem with Freedom ........................................ 181
Lesson 19 – Externalizing the Problem .......................................... 186

*Principle Six: Reconnecting with Your (Perfect) Weight* ............... 193
Lesson 20 – Weighty Issues-Determining Your Perfect Weight ... 193
Lesson 21 – Media Mayhem ........................................................... 204
Lesson 22 – Letting Go of Expectations ......................................... 205

*Principle Seven: Finding Your Happetite* ...................................... 209
Lesson 23 - Revisiting the Eating Continuum ............................... 209
Lesson 24 - Have You Ever Been a Normal Eater? ........................ 211
Lesson 25 - What's Your Plan: Structural or Observational? ....... 212
Lesson 26 - Nutrition Basics for Engaging Appetite ..................... 219
Lesson 27 - Making Friends with Your Happetite ........................ 228
Lesson 28 - Move Your Body .......................................................... 234
Lesson 29 - Moving Towards More Conscious Eating .................. 238

*The Nature of Recovery* .................................................................. 247

*References / Sources* ....................................................................... 257

*Appendix 1: DSM IV Criteria for Eating Disorders* ....................... 273

*Appendix 2: Monitoring Forms* ...................................................... 277

## Contents

*Appendix 3: Resources* ........................................................................ *281*

*Appendix 4: Getting Help If You Have an Eating Disorder* .............. *283*

*Appendix 5: Externalizing Activity/Venn Diagram* ......................... *285*

**Happetite** (hăep ə tīt), **n. 1.** Feeling, showing or expressing joy in one's instinctive physical desire for food or drink. **2.** Being happy and connected to one's appetite.

# *The Seven Principles of Happetite*

Everyone is born with a natural appetite. All babies know exactly what they need to eat. They know the quantity they need to eat and when. If your eating is no longer easy and natural, or if you have problems with food, eating or weight you have likely lost touch with your true appetite or what I like to call your happetite.

I wrote this book because I believe when you learn to listen to your natural and true appetite you will never have an eating problem again. You will also have a more enjoyable life.

Restrictive dieting isn't natural. Like plastic, it became commonplace in the last century and like plastic it hasn't been very healthy for the planet or her inhabitants.

For centuries, people listened to their bodies and ate according to their natural appetites. Dieting as we know it, only came about from around the 1850s as industrialisation gathered pace.

The word diet is derived from the Latin word diaeta and the Greek word diaita, meaning mode of living or diaitan meaning to direct one's own life. Our current cultural interpretation is far different and nearly always refers to specific allowances of food to control weight. Throughout this book the terms dieting and restrictive dieting will be used interchangeably to describe practices or systems of dieting for weight loss.

For all their efforts with dieting more than 30% of the industrialised world's population is overweight or obese and up to one in five college women in the U.S. have an eating disorder. There seems to be something terribly wrong with this picture.

You've heard this before but the bottom line is this: diets don't work. Every diet book ever published and every diet ever written was successful for the person who wrote it. Why then do so many of us have difficulty sticking with diets, or if we do stick with them, end up with obsessions around food and weight?

It's because dieting treats the symptoms, not the underlying causes. It's because we start trusting others more than we trust ourselves, and our own bodies. It's because we start trusting the food, eating, weight and shape rules of others more than our own inner guidance.

Many diets can teach us a lot about the food our bodies love best. Some diets help our bodies cope when we are sick. A low protein diet for the person with kidney disease, takes the pressure off the kidneys to cleanse their blood. It can delay the need for dialysis. A well-balanced carbohydrate intake helps someone with diabetes feel better by balancing their blood sugars.

But all too often diets are too restrictive and either set off the diet-binge cycle or trigger the starvation syndrome. The explosions afterward can be as debilitating as an exploding land mine.

I believe the current obsession with dieting and body image is a Westernised version of the ancient Chinese practice of footbinding. Dieting is as crippling to living a full life as footbinding was for ancient Chinese women.

Your body knows what is best for you to eat, how much to eat and when to eat – your job is to relearn how to listen to it. For example, many people think ice cream and chocolate are inherently bad. The truth is your body knows how much of those foods you can eat and when to eat them. Your body also knows how you will feel during and after eating them.

If you really wish to change your relationship to food you need to first examine who you are and identify the things that get in the way of your ability to listen and respond to your appetite.

In order to transform your experience, you will need to eliminate your current food, weight and shape rules.

The aim of this book is to help you first identify your eating problems and then take you through step-by-step to learn the principles, attitudes and skills needed to reconnect with your natural appetite. You will no longer be a prisoner of your immediate food cravings.

My vision is to help you live a life of freedom around food, eating, weight and shape. Your positive changes now will also have the benefit of impacting future generations.

### What's *Find Your Happetite* About?

This book is about giving you the tools and self-awareness to release yourself from the bondage of food and weight issues. There are seven principles that, if you work through them, will dramatically change your relationship to food. You literally won't know yourself.

In working with clients I have discovered three things that get in the way of your happetite and four things that move you towards your happetite.

What are the three things that get in the way of your happetite? What is limiting your ability to listen and respond to your natural appetite?

### 1) Physical Challenges

Physical ailments or issues may be preventing you from listening and responding to your natural appetite. These include hormonal, digestive and metabolic imbalances.

Having a strong metabolism and healthy digestion are crucial to maintaining your natural appetite. Disruption of these can strongly influence food cravings and how you eat. Hormonal issues, chemicals and pesticides, food allergies and intolerances also strongly influence how your bodies work and drive your appetites. You will begin to identify your individual physical challenges that prevent you from listening to your appetite and be given suggestions for solving those problems.

## 2) Emotional Barriers

Do you disconnect from your appetite and use food to medicate yourself when experiencing emotions? Are you an emotional eater? If you are struggling to understand and deal with emotional issues, you are destined for food and weight difficulties. Emotional barriers include using dieting or overeating to cope with unreleased or unprocessed emotions, 'feeling' fat (whether or not you are fat - because emotions are covered up by 'feeling' fat), and difficulties with understanding and dealing with a range of emotions. When you learn to work with underlying emotional barriers you are able to listen and respond to your natural appetite.

## 3) Mental Attitudes

Motivational issues fall into this category along with the negative beliefs and thoughts you have associated with weight, food and shape throughout your entire life. Making food decisions "from the neck up" prevents you from listening to your body. Challenging and overcoming these mental attitudes are crucial to finding your happetite.

What four things will help you listen and respond to your natural appetite?

## 1) Understanding Your Eating

To have freedom with food and weight issues you first will need to understand your current eating patterns. Principle One will help you answer the question: How do I eat without feeling the guilt and deprivation that goes hand-in-hand with dieting? *The Eating Continuum*™ describes various types of eating: eating disorders, disordered eating (including restrictive dieting), normal eating and conscious-choice eating and is discussed in detail along with the physical and psychological impact of the diet-binge cycle. The diet-binge cycle triggers the see-saw of emotions between guilt and deprivation, eventually leading to overeating, weight gain and constant ruminations about food and weight.

## 2) Understanding Your Happetite

Diets work for the short-term, but they do not help you figure out the answer to the question of what works in the long term. The whole notion of happetite is about transforming your eating and moving towards a more joyous state of living. This includes listening to your body and to your appetite. It's about self-acceptance. It's about reconnecting with your natural appetite. It's about having an understanding of the physiological and psychological reasons why diets don't work. Understanding all this will help you move towards appetite-driven eating.

## 3) Reconnecting with Your (Perfect) Weight

Let me define perfect weight: it is the weight your body wants to weigh, not a number that you have in your head. Take a deep breath. I know this is scary – you may say:
"I can't trust my body!"
"I have a target weight in mind."

# Find Your Happetite

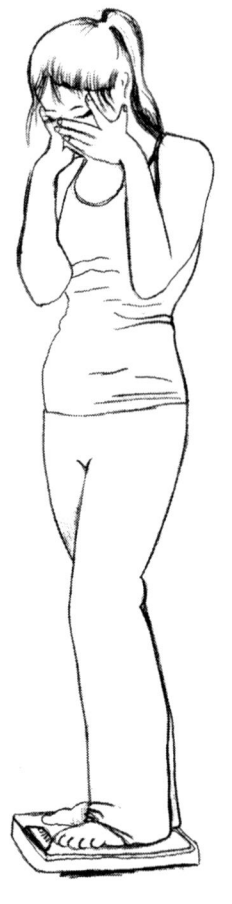

"I will not be happy until I weigh __."
"I hate that my body wants to weigh __."

Do you know what your natural weight is? Principle Six will help you figure out the answer to this question and then help you consider ways to reconnect with that weight. I promise if you stick with me through this chapter you will be surprised with the freedom and trust you can achieve. I promise you your body does NOT want to be carrying excess weight, even though there are plenty of stumbling blocks in our current food culture which make it difficult to find that natural weight.

You will also explore your weight history, your genetics and physiology. You will discover your body can be trusted. You will discover how the media influences the number you have in your head. You will explore how some food growing and manufacturing practices influence how your body uses food and increases the likelihood of the desire to overeat, and then diet. You will learn how to let go of expectations while still having an ability to make change.

## 4) Finding Your Happetite

Principle Seven is where you will bring all of your previous experience, experimenting and knowledge into formulating what will work in the long term. You will work out your own eating and weight management plan for life. You will learn to reconnect and be at peace with your natural weight and appetite, leading to a life free of weight, shape and food issues.

22

## The Nature of Recovery

The nature of recovery from food, eating, weight and shape issues is discussed in the last chapter. Recovery from any form of eating problem always involves transformation. Families who live with a child or teenager who has had an eating disorder are forever changed by the experience; people who come to terms with the food, eating, weight and shape issues that have plagued them are steadier and calmer in the face of other life difficulties. Ultimately *Find Your Happetite* is a spiritual journey because when you are intimately connecting, responding and trusting your appetite, you are intimately connecting with the whole of your body, mind and soul. When you are intimately connected with all these aspects of yourself in the physical realm (the physical, mental and emotional parts of your being) you are connected with who you really are.

In essence this book aims to help you become your own nutrition therapist. It is focused primarily on helping you find ways to manage your symptoms. It will also provide you with suggestions and references for seeking help for the underlying causes. You will need to deal with both symptoms and cause in order to find your happetite. I will be offering lots of ideas and suggestions but you will ultimately have to do the work.

By addressing your areas of blockage and resistance, you will open yourself to the potential for transformative change. The approach outlined has resulted in many positive changes for people who have the courage to challenge the cultural call to restrictively diet. You will be able to eat without guilt or deprivation, find freedom around food and no longer feel trapped. Your general wellbeing will also improve. *Find Your Happetite* is ultimately a life enhancement program.

This is a practical approach to the dilemma of food, weight and shape concerns. It is grounded in modern science and research: biology, biochemistry and psychology. There are lessons and experiments designed to help you help yourself. Instead of the experiments you might remember from high school when blowing up the Bunsen burner seemed like a good idea, these experiments will help you discover what works best for you.

Scientific information will be available for your rational mind, but in reality the intelligence of your own body is greater than all of the PhDs on the planet. There is no need to go off and read a few more articles on nutrition or get a science degree in order to eat more consciously. In fact, if you suddenly have the urge to do some research on weight management you will be better off having a lie down until the feeling passes. Seriously!

**The Experimental Approach**

The way you do the Happetite Training at the end of each chapter is crucial. I encourage you to be observant and curious. There is no 'right' or 'wrong' way to do the experiments to find your happetite. There is only your way, it is about whatever works for you! It's the 'take what fits and leave the rest' approach.

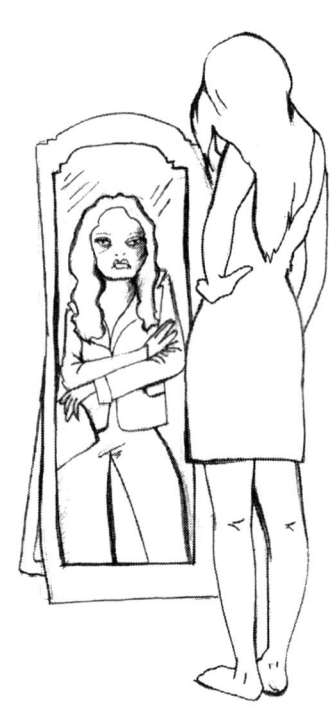

You should however be aware of the parts of you that will object to some of the things you are learning. These parts might be skeptical, plain rude or give you a really hard time. It can be helpful to give these parts a name like The Critic, The Body Bully, The Internal Terrorist, "It" or any other name that resonates for you.

Be aware when The Internal Terrorist is getting in the way of your curiosity. These parts of you will say things like:

"You shouldn't have that food you love because it will make you fat."

"You are too fat."

"You are a pig because you eat so much."

"You are hopeless because you can't ever follow diets."

"You are hopeless and worthless, too."

"Your thighs (or whatever body part you choose) are too big."

"You can't be trusted."

You might like to ask that part of you to step aside to allow your exploration while you read the book.

## Parts of You to Be Observant Of and Curious About

Tick one that applies to you:

____The Critic

____The Body Bully

____The Internal Terrorist ("IT")

____The Food and Weight Nazi

What other parts of you are you aware of, that are keeping you stuck in weight, food and eating dilemmas? Write them in the spaces below.

_____

_____

_____

## Parts of You to Choose For a Journey of Discovery

Tick one that appeals to you:

____The Adventurer

The adventurer part of you is about exploration, discovery and innovation.

____The Journalist

The journalist investigates and seeks out knowledge and experiences that supports your journey.

____The Reporter

This part of you observes and identifies 'what is' and reports about it.

____The Scientific Observer
The scientist classifies and analyses information gathered during objective observation.

____The Freedom Fighter
The freedom fighter causes change in a political or social order.

Any others?

_____

_____

_____

As we ate breakfast together after yoga one day, my friend Anne spoke about a way of being that she has found very helpful: having a high level of involvement in life but a low level of attachment to outcomes. That is what we are aiming for in this process. Look through the "glasses" or viewpoint of the positive part of you as you go through the exercises and experiments at the end of each chapter.

## How Have Your Concerns With Food, Eating, Weight and Shape Affected You?

The mental, physical, emotional and spiritual costs to a person in the prison of food and weight related concerns are enormous. Take a moment to think about how your own life has been affected by your dieting and concerns about eating, weight and shape:

- **Physical**

What physical costs have you experienced because of your concerns about food, eating, weight and shape? Examples include poor temperature regulation or constantly feeling cold, malnutrition leading to poor oral health, loss of menstruation due to low weight, difficulty with movement at either end of the spectrum of weight, hormonal imbalances from yo-yo dieting.

_____

_____

_____

- **Emotional**

What emotional costs have you experienced because of your concerns about food, eating, weight and shape? Examples include moodiness, depression, anxiety, and despair.

_____

_____

_____

- **Mental**

What mental costs have you experienced because of your concerns with food, eating, weight and shape? Examples include negative self-image, low self-esteem, and poor self-talk.

_____

_____

_____

- **Spiritual**

What spiritual costs have you experienced because of your concerns about food, eating, weight and shape? Examples include loss of hope, lack of joy and disconnection from the self including your higher self.*

_____

_____

_____

Restrictive dieting triggers each of these. And your autonomic nervous system moves you to act in dichotomous ways. Physically you either become numb or excess adrenaline increases anxiety to move you into "fight or flight". So if you are a binge eater you may numb out afterward in front of the television and fall asleep or the anxiety may trigger you to do some compulsive exercise or endlessly ruminate about what you have just eaten.

Mentally, you tend to have all or nothing thinking. You will either blank out or have a racing mind. Emotionally, you will alternate between guilt and deprivation, but eventually that

---

* The divine nature, universal mind, God, Yaweh, Source Energy, the Universe, the Infinite or however you experience "Oneness" or pure unconditional love.

escalates into fear of being fat or avoidance of situations involving food. Spiritually, you may become closed off to your spirituality and closed off to your higher self. Alternatively, you may walk around thinking you are elevating your consciousness by restrictively dieting and ignoring your appetite.

French philosopher Pierre Teilhard de Chardin famously said, "We are not human beings having a spiritual experience. We are spiritual beings having a human experience." Whether you believe that or not doesn't really matter. Detoxifying physically, emotionally and mentally will allow more joy and ultimately that is what we are all striving for as humans.

If you have been struggling with food, eating, weight and shape concerns for some time you may benefit from the support of a team skilled in treating eating and dieting issues. Many clinics offer team approaches or you can put together your own team. Ideally, each aspect (physical, emotional, mental and spiritual) will be addressed. You may find it helpful to speak with a skilled dietitian who incorporates a natural eating or non-dieting approach in their practice. You may also benefit from the help of other experts (such as physicians, clinical psychologists, physiotherapists, psychiatrists, social workers, counselors) and perhaps alternative practitioners to tackle the underlying causes.

In Appendix 3 there are resources and information on how to find people that may be able to help you. You can also go to www.findyourhappetite.com for more information.

**How Long Will It Take to Find My Happetite?**

The answer to the question of recovery time will vary depending on your motivation, your level of support, your commitment, focus and determination. In as little as a few weeks you may begin to notice a new level of freedom in your life around food and eating – but if it takes longer don't worry. It will depend on your ability to challenge your current view of yourself and our culture. It will depend on your willingness to explore the underlying causes to your current food, eating, weight and shape concerns. Once you make a clear decision to recover, transformation can sometimes be rapid. For other people it can take months or years. It helps if you can view the difficulties and setbacks you encounter during your recovery as signposts on the road to freedom. Each situation will give you information about how you use food, eating, weight and shape concerns to cope with other aspects of life and help you find other ways of being.

**My Story**

I recount the following personal story as a possibility, hoping that you too will find a way to move past externally-driven culturally-imposed ideals and find yourself at peace with food and eating, with your weight and shape. A step toward change can come about when you know you are not alone.

I'm a dietitian with a Master's Degree in counseling. I trained and worked as a Registered Dietitian (RD) in the U.S. for ten years before moving to Australia in 1992. I am now an Accredited Practicing Dietitian (the RD equivalent), and an Accredited Nutritionist working and living in Sydney.

I am a Nutrition Therapist, though a term I like better comes courtesy of my cheeky friend Martina: "psycho-dietitian". My expertise is in the area of symptom management for eating problems, in particular, eating disorders and in helping clients learn how to trust their bodies - and appetites - again. I work as part of a team and I also work one-on-one with clients and their families. I enjoy my work and find it very rewarding, but it wasn't always the case.

Even as a student I had my doubts about being a dietitian. I'd enrolled for the joy I found in helping others and in preparing, serving and eating nutritious food. Preparing food was a creative outlet for me, but the course work didn't seem to reflect what I'd hoped for.

Academically, however, I was up to the task so I stuck with it until my third year when I nearly dropped out midway. One of my clinical supervisors took me aside in a private meeting and said that I needed to lose weight because I didn't look like a dietitian. "What is a dietitian supposed to look like?" I silently thought to myself as shame crept furtively through my body... my mind wandered back to childhood:

I grew up on a family farm in Iowa, not far from where the Mississippi River slices through the glacier-leveled fields of the Mid-west. My five siblings and I were intimately connected with nature and the cycles of life. In the spring we helped Dad get the soil ready for planting corn, soybeans, and oats. We helped Mom with the garden. We'd cut out the 'eyes' of specially selected last-season potatoes and set them skin side up a few inches apart in newly dug holes in the black earth, or scatter tiny seeds of lettuce, spinach, carrots, cabbage, onion or melon in troughs along the rows of the garden. One of us would follow along with a hoe and instructions from Mom about how deep to cover the seeds. Every few years a new strawberry patch would be set out with the delicate green seedlings planted next to one another.

Before school each day we helped feed the cows, pigs and chickens that eventually provided our family with meat to eat. We helped with the twice daily milking and daily collection of eggs. We watched as the livestock gave birth to the new generation of pigs and calves. Through the summer months we helped with baling hay and weeding the garden. There was also the butchering of chickens, the ones that would feed us through the winter, thanks to the big deep freezer in the basement. (Butchering and plucking chickens was never a favorite task but one approached by all of us with alacrity and respect for the animals.) We watched during the hottest days of summer when the plants would literally shiver with growth. I'd sit with one of my brothers or sisters in the garden eating fresh fruit, peeling back the little paper lantern "coats" of the ground cherries before popping them directly into our mouths or picking raspberries off the spiky vines or sun-warmed apples off the tree. In the autumn we helped with the harvest and with preserving, canning and storing food to get us through the cold winter months.

Mealtimes were always family affairs. With eight of us in total there were never any short orders, we ate what we were given, or waited until the next meal or snack. We ate big breakfasts after morning chores, had hot lunches during the September-to-May school year or meals of sandwiches, homemade sweets and freshly made lemonade in the summer. There was always a snack in the afternoon and noisy meals before the evening milking. All the girls learned to cook from our mother, who was very adept in the kitchen. We ate to our appetites and never worried or thought much about eating, or weight, even though growing, harvesting, preparing and eating food was a big part of our life on the farm.

I brought myself back to the immediate conversation unfolding in the flourescent-lit room on campus. I felt the hot flush of humiliation as I sat in front of my professor. I'd always liked and admired her; I knew she had good intentions. I'm sure she only wanted the best for me and my career. And she was telling me I needed to lose weight. So my silent pondering of what a dietitian was supposed to look like was replaced with something much more judgmental, "There's something wrong with how I look and I'd better lose weight."

I had a strong connection to my natural appetite, but had not yet developed a strong sense of myself, or a healthy self-esteem, so I did what she suggested and I lost weight. Soon I started feeling physically and emotionally deprived and very quickly (and without much effort) regained the weight I'd lost, plus an extra kilogram or two. I felt a huge sense of guilt and failure. I also felt like a hypocrite (a dietitian that couldn't diet) and I lost track of the reason I'd enrolled in the course in the first place.

About that time I was diagnosed with a benign tumor in my jaw and had to have major surgery. I didn't make the connection between these two events back then but I do now. Being able to speak my truth and stand in personal integrity has been an on-going life challenge. Our physical body will always send us clues to our mental and emotional states if we pay attention.

Despite these setbacks I decided to finish the course and see what life would serve up. Even though I didn't 'look like a dietitian' I was allowed to graduate with my degree in dietetics. However, the events of that year weighed heavily on me during my first years of work, influencing my eating and prompting occasional halfhearted attempts to 'look like a dietitian' by dieting. Like any well-trained dietitian I could translate prescribed diets (for example an 1800 Kilocalorie low cholesterol diet) into a meal plan along with menu ideas. I understood food composition and could outline exactly what foods to eat during a day to fulfill the required Kilocalorie and nutrient needs *as understood by nutrition science at the time*. I highlight these words because anyone who reads scientific articles knows the only constant is change. Year-by-year various nutrients are touted as necessary for health and fitness – and others are put on the suspect list. The list of the do's and don'ts of nutrition fashion change as rapidly as clothing and accessories. At the time, polyunsaturated fats were the miracle cure (monounsaturated fats barely had a mention back then) and carbohydrates were to be avoided if you were any kind of fad diet aficionado. But no matter how scientific I was about what I wanted to eat, my appetite always won. I always ended up back at my normal weight.

On top of the influence of the apparent professional requirement to lose weight, I was yet to fully appreciate how early experiences in my life, both environmental and psychological, were playing out in the way I was with my body and with food. I've come to understand through my work, which the case studies in the book will highlight, that abuse exists and impacts our life in many ways, including food, eating, weight and shape issues. Alice Miller in *The Drama of the Gifted Child* says that all of us who grew up in the Western world grew up in abusive households. Having a higher standard of living than those that exist in third world nations does not exclude us from challenges to our psyche.

**Being a dietitian and dealing with these concerns created a level of internal conflict that eventually proved quite helpful. But first I had a lot of learning to do....**

One of my first jobs in the early 1980's was as a dietitian at a regional hospital in Wisconsin. I was assigned the task of working on a team (including physicians, nurses and psychiatrists) for a weight management program for the morbidly obese.

It was one of the first trials of the now ubiquitous liquid supplement dietary programs. The patients were put through a vigorous screening process and I was the dietitian in charge of the dietary protocols: Three liquid supplements a day until a state of ketosis ensued. (Ketosis is a medical term for a starved state that causes the muscles to be used for energy and shuts off the appetite. One of the telltale signs of ketosis is a sickly sweet smell to the breath.) Toward the end of the three-month protocol there was the addition of a small evening meal consisting mostly of animal-based protein. Eventually participants were weaned off the shakes and onto normal foods.

While weight loss results were dramatic, once patients started eating again many experienced rapid weight gain, and sometimes had episodes of binge eating. I was at a loss back then about how to help. I could easily empathise because of my own experience, with restrictive dieting in general and with a few weeks on the liquid supplement myself as a personal experiment, but I didn't know what to do or say to ease their distress.

Around this time I attended a workshop on natural eating by Ellyn Satter in Madison, Wisconsin. Ellyn is a registered dietitian and a licensed social worker. She is well known for her "division of duties" and recommendations for parents in regards to helping teach children how to eat. She suggests parents be responsible for what, when and where to eat, offering a wide variety of foods. Children are responsible for how much and whether they eat. She is also known for developing the Ellyn Satter Eating Competence Scale.

I remember standing at the back of the room during the afternoon and feeling a sense of "Ah-ha!" about what had been missing in my education: it was the role of normal eating and the pleasures of food. I also remember Ellyn telling the audience that by using the skills of normal eating, dietitians could have a container of ice cream in the shopping trolley without feeling hypocritical if they ran into a client at the supermarket. How strange that I'd been practicing as a dietitian for several years and hadn't reminded myself about the reason I'd become interested in the field of dietetics - to help others and to carry on my passion for food, cooking and eating.

Soon after this discovery, and with some effort on my part, my eating and weight started to normalise again. Within a year I'd enrolled in an educational counseling course at the University of

Wisconsin and started on-the-job training in the field of eating disorder treatment. My weight and clothing size has remained relatively stable for nearly 25 years since then. It took a little longer to accept and love the body that was lent to me for this life and there are some days where that is still a struggle, but by and large I can appreciate all the delights of the amazing machine that is my body. Though I won't ever be on the cover of Vogue, unless there are some radical changes to physical ideals in our Western culture, I can look in the mirror and see beauty. I hope after reading *Find Your Happetite* that you will too.

---

**My Commitment**

This is the day I make a commitment to my highest, wisest self to find the freedom that is my nature around food and weight concerns. I acknowledge that recovery may take some time, effort and investment. I am worth it. I deserve to live a life of freedom (and paradoxically gain control) around food, weight and shape.

Signature:                      Date:

## *Happetite Hints: Introduction*

**The key things that get in the way of finding your happetite:**
**Physical Challenges:** include, but are not limited to, hormonal, digestive and metabolic imbalances.
**Emotional Barriers:** such as unreleased or unprocessed emotions, 'feeling' fat (whether or not you are fat - because emotions are covered up by 'feeling' fat), and difficulties with understanding and dealing with a range of emotions.
**Mental Attitudes (Motivational Issues):** include lack of motivation along with the limiting beliefs and negative thoughts you have associated with weight, food and shape.

**The key things that move you towards finding your happetite:**
Understanding your current eating;
Understanding your happetite, or natural eating;
Reconnecting with your natural weight and
Finding your happetite.

**The experimental approach is crucial.** Aim to approach recovery as a journey of discovery.

**Be observant of and curious about the parts of you that are skeptical, rude or judgmental (the Critic, the Body Bully, the Internal Terrorist or others) and aim to use the parts of you that allow room for change and discovery (the Adventurer, Journalist, Reporter, Observer, Freedom Fighter or others).**

**Aim for a high level of involvement but a low level of attachment to outcomes.**

# *Principle One: Understanding Your Eating*

**Lesson 1: Understanding the Eating Continuum**

What is the Eating Continuum? It is a scale that describes various types of eating.

Eating disorders are often described as being on a continuum with Anorexia Nervosa on one end and Bulimia Nervosa on the other end, but the questions I always had in the back of my mind as I was working with clients was: "How can treatment move someone out of the cycle of disordered eating into normal appetite-driven eating, using the internal references they naturally had as children? How can they let go of the strong mental conditioning brought about by dieting and weight changes?"

The concept of the Eating Continuum has gradually evolved. The outer ends of the continuum fit the descriptions of diagnosable eating disorders as described by the American Psychiatric Association ICD (International Classification of Diseases) or the DSM-IV (Diagnostic and Statistical Manual IV). It also moves through restrictive dieting and overeating. Conscious-choice eating is in the middle of the continuum flanked on each side by normal appetite-driven eating.

## The Eating Continuum

| Anorexia Nervosa | Restricted Dieting | Restrained Eating | Normal Eating | Conscious-Choice Eating | Normal Eating | Over-eating | Binge eating | Bulimia Nervosa |
|---|---|---|---|---|---|---|---|---|
| | | | | *Appetite Driven Eating* | | | | |
| External References (Food Rules) | | | Internal References (No Food Rules) | | | External References (Food Rules) | | |

## Commentary on the Eating Continuum

Every person has their own particular eating style and all are functional:

Eating disorders are functional. Disordered eating is functional. Normal eating is functional. But some eating styles also create a lot of trouble physically, psychologically (emotional and mental issues) and spiritually. The difficulties that we experience when we're eating for reasons other than appetite may sometimes be difficult to let go. In order to move towards conscious-choice eating you must first accept where you're at on the continuum.

All of the disordered styles of eating (anorexia nervosa, restrictive dieting, restrained eating, overeating, binge eating and bulimia nervosa) are driven by external references such as

## Principle One: Understanding Your Eating

food rules, managing emotions or other reasons for eating or not eating, whether they are conscious or not, that are unrelated to appetite.

Finding your happetite means moving away from restrictive dieting. Most people need some help in letting go of long-standing patterns of restriction and overeating. For them some guidelines and/or a meal plan may be helpful. Later, in Principle Seven, I'll talk about who might benefit from these nutrition tools (Nutrition guidelines or a meal plan differ in important ways from restrictive dieting). The next diagram shows where Guidelines or a Meal Plan fit onto The Eating Continuum.

| Anorexia Nervosa | Restricted Dieting | Restrained Eating | Guidelines or Meal Plan | Normal Eating | Conscious Choice Eating | Normal Eating | Guidelines or Meal Plan | Over-eating | Binge eating | Bulimia Nervosa |
|---|---|---|---|---|---|---|---|---|---|---|
| External References (Food Rules) ||| | *Appetite Driven Eating* <br><br> Internal References (No Food Rules) ||||| External References (Food Rules) |||

Normal eating is appetite-driven. It may also have other factors influencing it such as social situations, family background, cultural and religious influences, but it is mostly driven by an internal reference e.g. "How hungry am I?" and "What am I hungry for?"

Conscious-choice eating has less to do with societal structures and much more to do with what is good for you, your body, and the planet. Conscious-choice eating fits in with your values. It is different from restrictive dieting in so many ways. When you are making food choices and eating from a place of conscious choice you have freedom around food, your eating is natural, you are not driven by guilt if you do eat, or deprivation if you don't, and you have a harmonious relationship with yourself and your body.

**Is This Book Useful For Someone with an Eating Disorder?**

As someone recovers from an eating disorder they will naturally pass through each phase of the continuum. This book will be most useful towards the end of recovery when treatment is about re-learning how to respond to one's natural appetite. Because of the complex nature of eating disorder treatment, this book will focus on the other parts of the continuum rather than treatment of diagnosable eating disorders. Many of the case studies will feature clients who have recovered from an eating disorder with details about how they were able to move to more normal eating during the latter stages of recovery.

**Descriptions of Phases of the Continuum**

The following descriptions are based on my clinical experience and observation*. (Diagnostic criteria for eating disorders from the Diagnostic and Statistical Manual IV using evidence-based research is included in Appendix 1.)

---

* Clinical observation is a subjective form of evaluation. Evidence-based research refers to the use of systematic empirical research and scientific studies (the best being randomised control trials), as a base for determining best practices. Since the 1990s evidence-based practice seeks the use of treatments that show significant effectiveness for specific problems.

Principle One: Understanding Your Eating

## Eating Disorders Including Anorexia Nervosa, Bulimia Nervosa, Eating Disorders Not Otherwise Specified and Binge Eating Disorder

- ❑ You spend 75% of the day or more thinking about food, weight and shape.
- ❑ You are defensive of, or secretive about, your eating and compulsive activities. You notice your eating is very different from how you ate when you were young. The "eating disorder" and "the self" are difficult to separate and feel as if they are one.
- ❑ You find almost anything can trigger eating disordered thoughts, even a simple "How are you?" is interpreted by the eating disordered part of you as "I am fat and worthless."
- ❑ Compulsive activities are the norm - exercising to the point of exhaustion or injury, restrictive eating, avoiding certain foods, bingeing and purging. This may also include obsessive cleaning, washing hands, alcohol and drug use, etc...
- ❑ If you are not engaging in your chosen compulsive activities you feel fear and anxiety; your life is structured in an attempt to manage these and other feelings.
- ❑ You either have daily emotional outbursts around food, weight and shape issues or are emotionally shut down and numb to your world.
- ❑ Your efforts to seek control sometimes end in control and sometimes end in chaos. You may seek control by following routines and structure.
- ❑ You have loved ones expressing concern and putting demands on you; you feel isolated and separate yourself from the people you used to feel close to.
- ❑ Your health is compromised in significant ways.
- ❑ In the early stages you may be in denial about how the illness is affecting your life.

## Restrictive Dieting, Restrained Eating, Under-Eating, Over-Eating or Binge Behaviors

- ❑ You spend up to 75% of your day judgmentally thinking about food, eating, weight and shape.

- ❏ Your eating is very different from how you ate when you weren't concerned about food, weight and shape. In other words, different from when you last ate normally, ate according to your appetite or before you first started dieting. Some people have had food, weight and shape concerns for as long as they can remember.
- ❏ You are able to separate "the disordered eating part" of you from "the self". In other words you can see chunks of who you really are when the disordered eating isn't present.
- ❏ The disordered eating part of you is triggered at times and you are aware enough to manage the triggers some of the time.
- ❏ Your eating is often followed by feelings of guilt, or you feel deprived if you don't eat.
- ❏ Compulsive activities still feature but you are aware of them and are aiming to manage them. You may be taking a course of action, other than dieting, to manage the compulsions.
- ❏ Your efforts to seek control sometimes end in control and sometimes end in chaos. You usually seek control by following routines and structure; this is less overt and obsessive than when eating disorders are present.
- ❏ Emotions may be 'stuck' in your physical body. When they are released through physical activity or bodywork you may re-experience some of the emotions leading to a sense of feeling out of control again. You will make an effort to manage those emotions in some way.

## **Normal Eating**
- ❏ Less than 10% of your day is spent thinking about food, weight and shape issues. The thinking is based on self-care rather than criticism; it is observational rather than judgmental.
- ❏ Your eating is mostly driven by appetite.
- ❏ You are aware and understand how at times you may try to manage your health (and perhaps your life) by attempting to control your food, weight and shape.

## Principle One: Understanding Your Eating

- ❑ You may be conscious of the nutritional values of foods and just as likely you may choose foods based solely on taste with no regard to nutritional value.
- ❑ You may eat regular meals and snacks or you may graze on foods throughout the day depending on your appetite, the availability of food, work schedule, social schedule and other factors.
- ❑ Your eating is not driven by guilt or deprivation.

*"With my injury and not being able to exercise I would have dieted and binged. I've seen that I can eat normally, have a life and not gain huge amounts of weight."*
-L.M. Client

### **Conscious-Choice Eating/Deliberate Eating**
- ❑ Your eating is driven by appetite, the internal references of hunger and satiety and other internal cues.
- ❑ You make conscious food choices based on nutrition, the life force* of food, and how food impacts your physical body and the planet.
- ❑ Your choices may include not acting on impulses to eat.
- ❑ You make food choices intuitively, independent of other factors such as work schedule and social schedule.
- ❑ Your eating is almost effortless and your food choices do not trigger either the starvation syndrome or the diet-binge cycle.
- ❑ Your eating and food choices are in alignment with your core values and are self-nurturing.

---

* In scientific terms this relates, in part, to the enzymatic properties found in food.

"You know these questions of yours as to what, when and how much a person should eat – they are best answered by the individual's own body. The sensations of hunger and thirst are designed to send a signal to each particular individual, indicating when he should take in food. This precise moment is the right one for each person. The world of technocracy being incapable of affording each individual the opportunity of satisfying his hunger and thirst at the moment desired by his body has tried to force him into it's own schedule based on nothing but this world's own helplessness, and then attempted to justify this compulsion in the name of some sort of efficiency...Man should take in food at the moment advised by his body and there can be no other advisor."

*- From The Ringing Cedars of Russia, Book 1 "Anastasia"*

## Principle One: Understanding Your Eating

One would think eating to your appetite would happen naturally; it should be as simple as breathing. But due to the overlying concerns and issues that amass during the course of a life it can become difficult to listen and respond to your natural appetite.

**In Practice**

I work as part of a multidisciplinary team at the Meridian Clinic at Total Health Care. It is an eating disorders outpatient clinic and our team includes a pediatrician, social worker and physiotherapist. When clients come to see us they are usually at either end of the continuum, with diagnosable eating disorders. Assessment and treatment of eating disorders is often complicated. Diagnosis may have been delayed by months or years because other confounding problems have been disguising the eating disorder as digestive or metabolic conditions. Psychological and physiological (medical and nutritional) problems intersect making a cohesive treatment plan essential. As recovery ensues some of the most challenging parts of treatment for clients are around letting go of eating disordered thoughts (negative thoughts about food, eating, weight and shape). Moving into appetite driven eating by trusting one's body can be confronting, challenging and liberating!

## Happetite Training

<u>Exercise One:</u>

Have a look at the Eating Continuum below. Read the descriptions of the various styles of eating on pages 41-43 and tick the boxes that apply to you. Put an (x) on the continuum that best represents your attitudes and behaviors today.

| Anorexia Nervosa / Restricted Dieting / Restrained Eating | Normal Eating / Conscious Choice Eating / Normal Eating | Over-eating / Binge eating / Bulimia Nervosa |
|---|---|---|
| | ***Appetite Driven Eating*** | |
| External References (Food Rules) | Internal References (No Food Rules) | External References (Food Rules) |

## Principle One: Understanding Your Eating

Exercise Two:

Step 1. Think about other times in your life - as a child and adolescent, as a single person, married or living in shared accommodation, other times - where were you on the Eating Continuum then? Take note of when you have been a normal or conscious-choice eater. When was the last time you had no concerns about food, eating, weight or shape? Note your answers:

_____

_____

_____

Step 2. Write a statement describing your current situation and way of being in regards to food, weight and shape. For example it might go something like this: 'I feel unhappy about how I look most of the time and I feel stuck in the diet-binge cycle.'

_____

_____

_____

_____

Step 3. Now write out a vision for your eating and way of being in regards to food, weight and shape. Write it as if you are already experiencing that way of being and keep the focus on how you feel rather than on a specific weight. For example 'I am content with my weight and shape. I am so happy to have freedom around food and to feel connected to my appetite.' Use some of the statements describing normal and conscious-choice eating. Rewrite your vision and place it where you can reread it often.

The vision I have for myself is:

_____

_____

_____

_____

_____

Exercise Three:

If you think you have an eating disorder, in other words you marked an (x) at either end of the continuum and are currently not in treatment then I strongly encourage you to search Appendix 4 or your local Yellow Pages for a list of treatment centers and resources. Pick up the phone today. Experiment until you find appropriate treatment for your situation.

This book will help later on, but in the early stages you will need strong support and containment of your eating disordered behaviors. Having a proper assessment and finding treatment now will significantly improve and shorten your time in recovery.

Here is how one client described her recovery:

"Having anorexia is like living with your eyes closed. All you can do is struggle in the dark on your own, trying to find your way with only the darkness to guide you. It wasn't until I opened my eyes that I could start to see myself and the world around me clearly, even though I didn't always like the things I saw, at least my eyes were open and they were my own."

## Lesson 2: Self-Acceptance

*"Nothing in the world has ever changed by railing against it. Things only change when we become aware and accept what is."*
-Echart Tolle

This lesson is about being okay with wherever you are on the eating continuum and with your eating, weight and shape. That is easy to say but hard to practice. It's easy to accept the parts of ourselves that we love, but difficult to accept the shadowy parts that challenge us, make life difficult and prompt negative feelings such as shame, embarrassment, self-loathing and despair.

How do you move in the direction of normal or conscious-choice eating? Do you have a vision of being able to listen to your appetite, but come unstuck when you are asked to begin accepting your body and current behaviours? Does the fear of weight gain re-emerge? Does it prompt thoughts of wanting to diet again? Do you want to make better choices, but find the feelings of disgust with your weight and food choices overwhelm and trap you? Do you feel out of control? Do you feel hopeless about ever getting out of the cycle?

Progress through recovery relies on your ability to accept yourself and your behaviours. By accepting your current situation you paradoxically move into a position where change is possible. What would it take for you to accept your current situation?

## Commentary on Self-Acceptance

Acceptance of where you are on the continuum is crucial in order to move towards more conscious-choice eating. One of the terms that we use in treatment is "radical acceptance". This isn't to say that you have to resign yourself to the current state of your life forever, but it is to acknowledge that where you are is "perfect" for right now.

*"Denial ain't just a river in Egypt."*
–Mark Twain

One of the ways to move towards acceptance is with the use of mindfulness. Mindfulness is an ancient practice found in many Eastern philosophies including Buddhism, Taoism and Yoga. It has been more recently used in western psychology and is increasingly recognised as an effective way to reduce stress, increase self awareness, enhance emotional intelligence and open up to new ways of feeling, thinking and acting.

Jon Kabat-Zinn, one of the leading authorities on the use of mindfulness defines it this way: "Paying attention in a particular way: on purpose, in the present moment and non-judgmentally."

Mindfulness involves consciously bringing awareness to your current experience with openness, interest and receptiveness. It is about waking up to ourselves and appreciating wherever we are in each moment. Kabat-Zinn calls it "the art of conscious living."

Acceptance and Commitment Therapy (ACT) uses mindfulness as one of its practices. ACT does not aim to reduce the symptoms, but rather "transform our relationship with our difficult thoughts and feelings so that we no longer perceive them as symptoms, instead we learn to perceive them as harmless even if uncomfortable transient psychological events."

A beautiful allegorical tale relating to this task is told in the film "Avatar". The lead character Jake Sully, as avatar, must choose and bond with a bird/beast, one of the Ikran or mountain banshees. (In Irish folklore the banshee is a female spirit who wails and cries, warning of impending death.) The banshee must also choose Jake. But first the bird/beast banshee tries to kill Jake, as all shadow-selves do. Jake struggles with the banshee he has chosen, while others look on expecting him to die, but Jake eventually mounts the neck of the bird and bonds with it. However the test is not yet over. The beast is so powerful that at first Jake rides it in an uncontrollable way, nearly coming off the banshee with every flap of its wings. Jake is quickly propelled into potency, learning to direct the beast with his pure focus of intention. Just as Jake struggles with the banshee, we struggle with our negative thoughts and feelings until we see the lessons in them and gain strength and wisdom from our experiences.

## Principle One: Understanding Your Eating

**In Practice**
**Ally**

Ally* was referred by a psychotherapist for help in challenging her ongoing binge eating behavior. She'd had an eating disorder of one form or another for 16 years. Early on it was anorexia, followed by 11 years of bulimia nervosa. She finally stopped purging (vomiting) a couple of years ago.

I was curious during her assessment; I asked how she managed to stop the purging behavior after using it as a coping skill for so long. "I stopped giving myself a hard time," was her reply.

She used self-acceptance to help transform her experience. She was able to give up the purging behavior because she could allow herself to see it as the coping skill it was. In part, along with therapy and symptom management, her compassionate stance of acceptance allowed her to move forward.

---

* Throughout the book names, ages and other identifying features have been changed for confidentiality. Some of the "In Practice" case studies are composites of several clients.

## Happetite Training

Exercise Four:

See if you can identify some of the destructive emotions, thoughts and actions you have around food, eating, and weight. Use one of the monitoring sheets in Appendix 2. Start with monitoring events for one day. Take note of where you give yourself a hard time. Now comes the interesting part. See if you can move into a space of acceptance. Just like Ally did in the previous example. How would you talk with yourself if you viewed yourself as your best friend? For example you might say to yourself, "I see how you have used this to cope and I'm so glad you're now willing to find someone to help."

Exercise Five:

Practice being mindful when you are doing a daily activity. For example brushing your teeth or making a drink. My friend Fiona and I recently discovered we both do this when we are making our morning coffee. Here's one version of mindfulness while making coffee:

I gather the three parts of my little stovetop espresso machine and think of the lovely time I had finding this little pot during a trip to Melbourne to visit my Italian friend Sandra. She took me to a beautiful little deli on Brunswick Street and spoke in Italian to the proprietor and eventually, with knowing nods and smiles all around, they presented me with this particular espresso machine which I purchased pronto.

While looking out my window and giving thanks for the morning, I gather the milk, honey, coffee beans and grinder and I take out a little pot for heating the milk. I think of all the people all over the world who have contributed to this moment. The coffee plantation workers in Guatemala or Papua New Guinea, the bees that have created the honey and the workers who have harvested and packed it. As I grind the beans, I allow the senses to open up and experience the smell, sound, sight, touch and eventually taste. That first sip is like the first sip of coffee I've ever taken. I am curious. The taste is always different. Most mornings I will sit on my balcony with my pooch at my feet or on my lap, drinking my coffee in silence and watching the insects and birds as they get on with their day in the beautiful green treetops that surround me. Some mornings I'm distracted and I don't enjoy the coffee nearly as much as when I am being mindful. Not once do I think about the nutritional benefits. Coffee satisfies every sense and I have great joy in that one cup a day. A few times a week I take a similar approach when I make fresh juice. Now if I could just take this approach with everything I do…

Here's how mindfulness works for my friend Mary Kay Aide (www.spaforyoursoul.com):

> "I chose sweeping the floors. My house is all hardwood floors. I have two kids, two cats and a dog, so my floors need sweeping a lot (I mean a LOT!). Originally, my sweeping habits were tense, frenzied affairs. Sometimes I would try to sweep while talking on the phone, picking up things as I went along, having conversations with the kids or just grumbling about all the dust and animal hair in my house. Not very relaxing. Now, when I pick up a broom, I take a deep breath and slow down my breathing. I pay attention to the feel of the broom in my hand, the subtle changes in my muscles in my arms and upper back as I sweep. I notice the sound of the bristles against the floor and I notice the results as I sweep a room. It's amazing how relaxing that time is and I've noticed that the response has become automatic whenever I pick up a broom. Believe it or not, I really enjoy sweeping! Who knew?"

## Lesson 3: Understanding the Cycle of Restriction and Overeating (Diet - Binge Cycle)

*'You can't do what you want, till you know what you are doing.'*
*-Moshe Feldenkraus*

Restrictive dieting generally leads to one of two pathways. Both pathways prompt physiological and psychological difficulties:

### Pathway One: The Diet-Binge Cycle

Restriction → feeling deprived physically and emotionally → getting trapped in the diet-binge cycle → challenges to metabolic, digestive and hormonal systems and one's psyche.

Principle One: Understanding Your Eating

*Pathway Two: The Starvation Syndrome*

Restriction → leading to muscle wasting and appetite shut-off → the starvation syndrome → challenges to metabolic, digestive and hormonal systems and one's psyche.

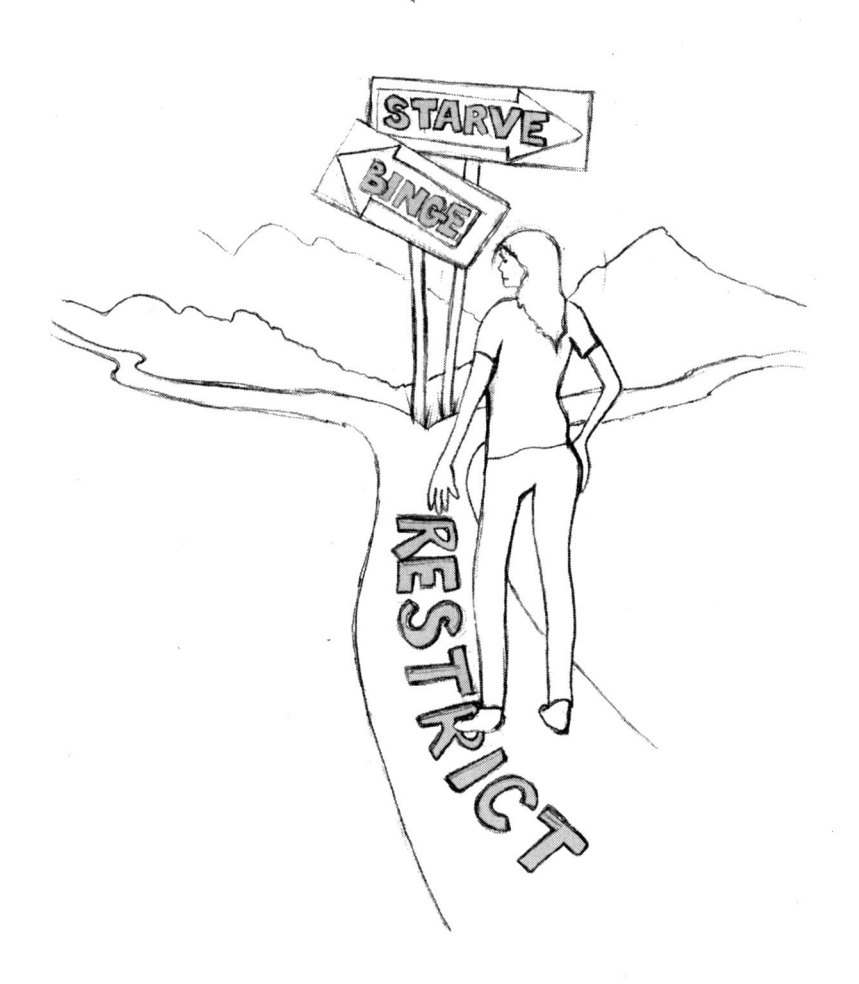

The rest of this chapter will explore Pathway One in detail. Later, in Principle Three, the starvation syndrome will be explored.

## Commentary on Understanding the Cycle of Restriction and Overeating (Diet-Binge Cycle)

Restrictive dieting - even thinking you should be dieting in order to lose weight but not actively restricting your food intake - leads to feelings of emotional and physical deprivation, and eventually overeating. Restrictive dieting leads to overeating, and possibly bingeing, which leads to more dieting, and more overeating. The pendulum swings wider and wider.

The more you restrict your eating the more you eventually overeat or binge. The tighter you pull the pendulum, the more forcefully it swings back. Once in the cycle, the thoughts and behaviours around food, eating, weight and shape become all-consuming. Understanding the diet-binge cycle is fundamental to moving towards more conscious choices with your eating.

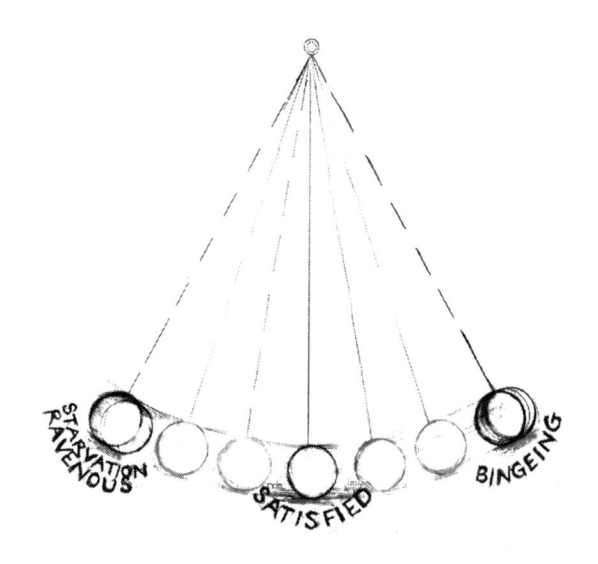

The cycle can start anywhere on the wheel depicted on the next page, but for the sake of this discussion let's start with what you say to yourself when you look in the mirror. Think about it right now, what was the first thing that came to your mind when you looked in the mirror this morning? Did you think, "I'm beautiful" or some other statement of positive regard? Or was it, "I'm fat and ugly" or some other negative adjective? Was it a generalised thought or more specific judgments? Typically the diet-binge cycle is triggered and perpetuated by powerful negative thoughts or by standing on the scales and giving your weight some negative meaning.

Principle One: Understanding Your Eating

# The Diet/Binge Cycle

(This cycle may vary from person to person)

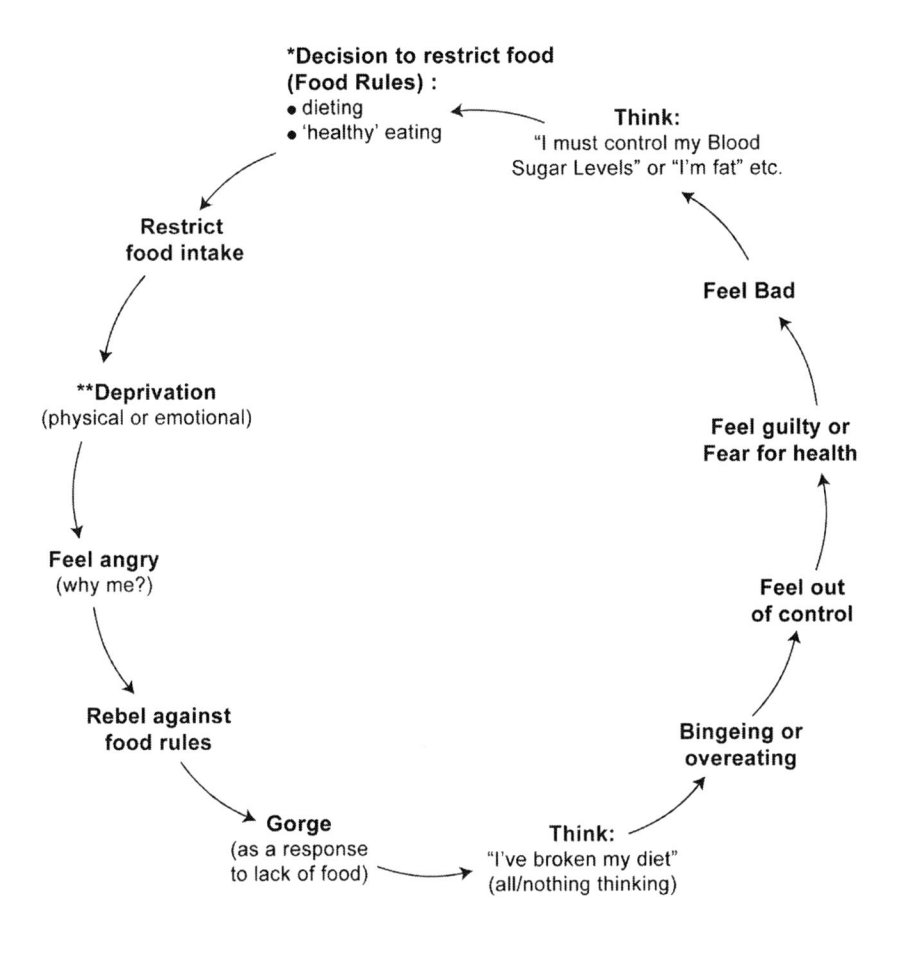

*Decision to restrict food
(Food Rules):
- dieting
- 'healthy' eating

Think:
"I must control my Blood Sugar Levels" or "I'm fat" etc.

Feel Bad

Restrict food intake

Feel guilty or Fear for health

**Deprivation
(physical or emotional)

Feel out of control

Feel angry
(why me?)

Bingeing or overeating

Rebel against food rules

Gorge
(as a response to lack of food)

Think:
"I've broken my diet"
(all/nothing thinking)

\* Can be self-imposed or imposed by health professional

"Shoulds" and "Should nots" develop

Cycles adapted from Anti-Diet:
You Are Not What You Eat: by B.J. Coish. 1988

\*\* Emotional deprivation
  - from not eating for comfort

\*\* Physical deprivation
  - lower metabolism
  - increases body's ability to absorb food
  - increases drive to eat and food pre-occupation

The next step of this cycle is making a decision about what kind of action to take in response to those thoughts. In particular, if you think you need to change your weight or shape in some way there will be some decision around food intake. Here's where food rules show up. There are a variety of ways this is interpreted depending on your dieting history. You could have food rules around:

- Eating *only* healthy foods;
- Avoiding eating. "Yesterday was so bad I'm not going to eat today.";
- Avoiding certain foods or food groups. (Avoiding fat or avoiding foods with sugar or avoiding products that contain white flour.);
- Avoiding groups of foods for ecological or religious reasons. (If these avoidances are imposed upon you and are not 'internally motivated' they can still trigger the diet-binge cycle.);
- Following a strict diet – e.g. the latest celebrity diet or one of the hundreds advertised each year; or
- Counting calories, counting grams of fat or counting anything.

Restricting food or just thinking you *should* be restricting food, are both a result of *thinking you need to lose weight* or that there is something wrong in some way. Perhaps you have had a recent health scare or your partner has made a comment about your body. Thinking you need to lose weight is the main driver behind the diet-binge cycle. **Whether or not you actually restrict food or follow through with the decisions you make about how to eat seems not to make any difference to the continuation of the cycle.** This is a subtle but potent distinction. It is a mental decision based on a deficit: that you are fat or need to lose weight. It is a mental decision to restrict because there is something *wrong* rather than coming from a place of conscious-choice and self-care. You may be fat but thinking that will only make you fatter, because whether or not you restrict your food intake, you will still end up feeling deprived physically and emotionally. And the diet-binge cycle is in motion. This is why it is so essential to start taking a different approach.

> *"Insanity: doing the same thing over and over again and expecting different results."*
> -Albert Einstein

The diet-binge cycle triggers strong responses. Physically you can feel deprived because your body is lacking the nutrients and energy that it needs to get through the day. Emotionally you might be deprived because you aren't getting a food that satisfies you on some other level. For example, you may associate certain foods with nurturing. It might be something that your mother fed you when you were little and still unconsciously makes you feel nurtured. Denying your self either physically or psychologically sets you up for food cravings. Cravings are a big red flag that some physical, emotional or mental need is not being met.

Next on the cycle come the strong feelings of frustration. You might ask yourself the questions: Why me? Why am I stuck in this situation? It's the inner child in us having a tantrum against being told 'no': "No, you can't eat what you want, you are not deserving of satisfying that unmet need".

Further along in this cycle we start to rebel against those food rules. It is the inner adolescent now saying, "I can do what I want!" We break the food rules initially in response to lack of food, the red flag from our body is that we need more food. Carbohydrates such as cereal, bread, biscuits and sugary foods are commonly eaten at this stage of the cycle for the quick boost they give to our lagging blood sugars. Next in the cycle is what is termed "all-or-nothing thinking". You might say something like this to yourself, "I promised myself I wouldn't eat until dinner, it is only 4 pm and I've broken my promise. I'm hopeless anyway, so I may as well keep eating." Bingeing starts - psychologically-driven overeating. You feel out of control. If you are suffering from an eating disorder, you may take steps to stop feeling out of control after bingeing. Vomiting, use of laxatives or exercising compulsively all help relieve the stress and anxiety of bingeing. So, no matter what, you always end up feeling bad, feeling overwhelmed with guilt, feeling hopeless and helpless and the cycle starts over. You think there is something wrong with you, when in fact you are simply trapped in a cycle that prevents you from listening to your natural appetite

Overeating is sometimes referred to as disinhibited eating and dieting is called 'high dietary restraint'. Sometimes we learn these "skills" from our parents and pass them on to the next generation ourselves.

Restrictive dieting leads to overeating, always. Several studies show that restrictive dieting is the most commonly recognised risk factor for any disorder of eating. The risk for dieters to develop an eating disorder is up to eight times higher than that for non-dieters.

Research suggests you are at a higher risk of undertaking restrictive dieting if you have:
- Low self-esteem
- Body dissatisfaction
- Depression
- High body weight
- Social anxiety or
- Have an external locus of control - the belief that others, fate or chance primarily determine events.

Over and over again studies confirm that people want to lose weight, even when they are already in a healthy weight range, and that use of weight loss behaviors is often related to a desire to be thin rather than healthy.

I want to emphasise again, that *whether or not you are actively dieting it is the desire to lose weight that drives the diet-binge cycle.*

## In Practice
### Jim
Jim, a 46-year old community worker, described his problem as compulsive eating. He did not binge but ate foods such as biscuits and soft drinks, which he thought he shouldn't be eating. By keeping food and mood records he discovered that his overeating

occurred mostly in the middle of the night and was related to feelings of depression, anxiety, sadness, shame and worthlessness.

Jim's daytime pattern of eating was reasonably normal. He generally ate three meals and two or three snacks a day and included a wide variety of foods. On assessment his height was 175 centimetres and his weight was 92 kilograms, giving him a Body Mass Index (BMI) of 30. BMI is a commonly used statistical measure of body weight based on a person's weight and height.

His highest weight was his current weight of 92 kilograms and he had a low weight of somewhere between 68-70 kilograms at age 20 and after periods of restrictive dieting. His reference weight* was somewhere in the range of 61-77 kilograms,

Our discussions focused on the "shoulds" that he carried with him regarding his eating and weight and how this kept him in the restriction and overeating cycle, despite the fact he hadn't *actually* dieted in more than a decade. By dealing with the underlying emotional drivers with a therapist and challenging what he thought he should be eating, he was able to normalise his eating and his weight over a number of months.

**Lois**

Lois was a 20-year old media student who reported a 10-year history of bingeing and chronic dieting. She remembered overeating from as young as six, blaming lots of takeaway foods for her regularly increasing weight. She first became conscious of her weight at 13, when she weighed 75 kilograms. Her first diet was at age 16. She reports losing 20 kilograms four or more times since age 16, about once every year. She described herself as an emotional and stress eater. Her highest previous weight had been 78 kilograms, her lowest 55 kilograms was at age 17 after she had been on a Weight Watchers program for some time. At assessment her weight was 61 kilograms. Her BMI was 24 and she had a reference range of 51-64 kilograms (BMI 20-25).

---

* Reference weight in this instance was determined by using the BMI 20-25. The issue of reference weights and BMI will be explored in detail in Principle Six.

Lois weighed herself three or four times a week, had been compulsive about exercise in the past and had described recent erratic eating at the time of assessment. She had many dieting beliefs and food rules. She always planned to eat three meals a day, but when she got hungry between meals she tended to binge.

She reported drinking very little each day, usually just two caffeinated drinks.

She told me she would like to weigh 50-55 kilograms. She eventually agreed that even though that weight was within her reference range it was unrealistic given her current weight and her weight history. She had only been able to get to 55 kilograms by being very restrictive with her eating in the past.

My sessions with Lois focused on breaking the diet-binge cycle by establishing a pattern of more regular eating and increasing her fluid. (Many people live with chronic dehydration and if any one thing can help your cells work better it's making sure you're drinking adequate amounts of hydrating fluids throughout the day. 'Adequate' is 35-45 ml fluid per kilogram of body weight; for most people this equates to about 1.5 – 2 litres fluid per day, the equivalent of six to eight 250 ml glasses. You will require more if it is hot or your activity prompts lots of sweating.)

As part of her nutrition plan Lois agreed to stop weighing herself. Initially she aimed to weigh herself just once a week at home and then less frequently until she was more detached about her weight and trusting of her body.

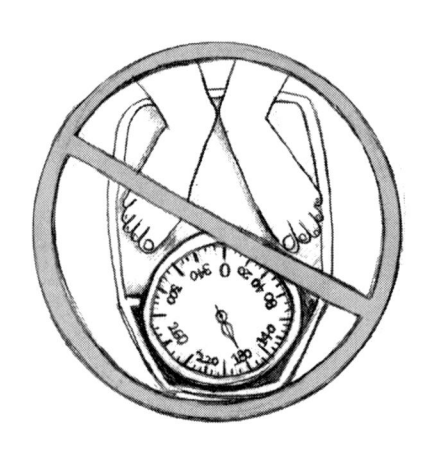

She also kept food and mood records making links between her eating and her mood. She experimented with having three meals and three snacks a day and including fluids at mealtimes. She also enlisted support from her mother, whom she lived with, to help with meal preparation and eating normal meals with her.

Principle One: Understanding Your Eating

## Happetite Training

Exercise Six:

Make a list of your "shoulds" and "shouldn'ts" involving food, weight and shape.

Exercise Seven:

Use The Diet-Binge Cycle Worksheet on the next page, answering the questions and writing in *your own* particular thoughts, words and phrases about *your* food rules, emotions and actions as you have experienced them when you were in the diet -binge cycle. Remember that even if you haven't restrictively dieted, if you believe you *should* be losing weight you may still be in the cycle.

# The Diet/Binge Cycle Worksheet

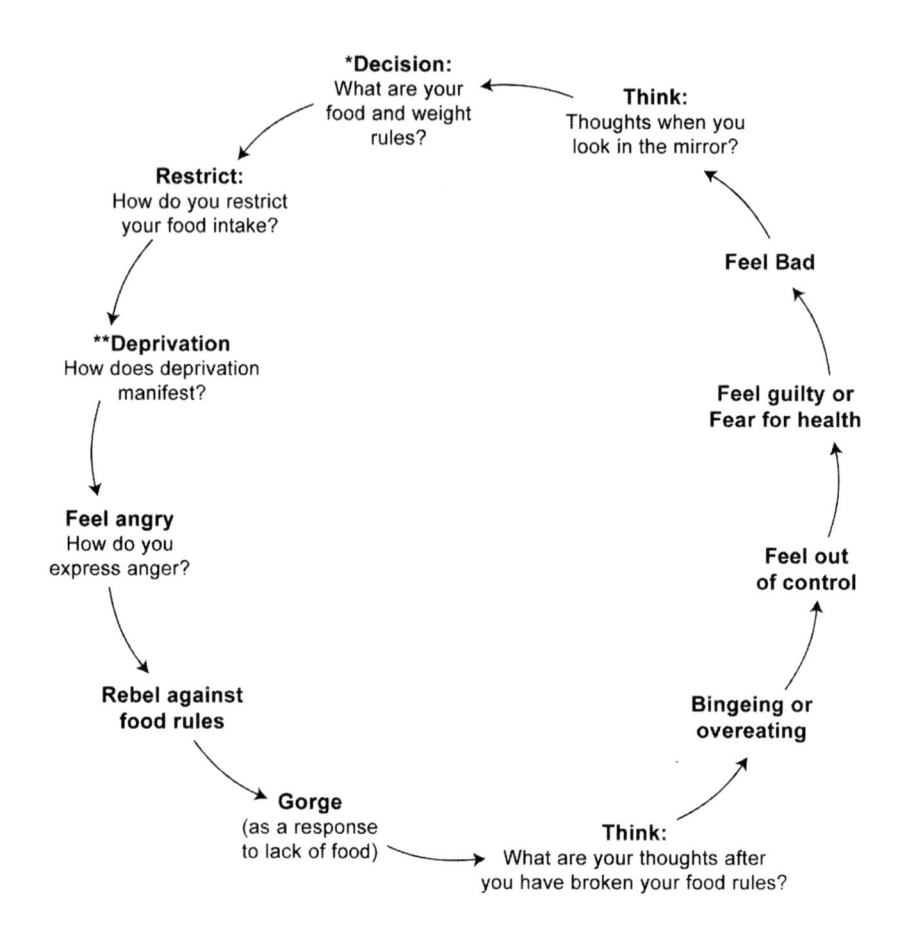

**\*Decision:** What are your food and weight rules?

**Think:** Thoughts when you look in the mirror?

**Restrict:** How do you restrict your food intake?

**Feel Bad**

**\*\*Deprivation** How does deprivation manifest?

**Feel guilty or Fear for health**

**Feel angry** How do you express anger?

**Feel out of control**

**Rebel against food rules**

**Bingeing or overeating**

**Gorge** (as a response to lack of food)

**Think:** What are your thoughts after you have broken your food rules?

\* Can be self-imposed or imposed by health professional

"Shoulds" and "Should nots" develop

Cycles adapted from Anti-Diet: You Are Not What You Eat: by B.J. Coish. 1988

\*\* Emotional deprivation
- from not eating for comfort

\*\* Physical deprivation
- lower metabolism
- increases body's ability to absorb food
- increases drive to eat and food pre-occupation

Principle One: Understanding Your Eating

Exercise Eight:

Fill in the worksheet on page 66.

In the first column write a list of all the diets and weight loss methods you have tried or experimented with in your life. Include those times when you thought you *should* be dieting but didn't actively restrict your intake.

In the second column note the age you were when you were attempting to lose weight with that particular approach. In the third column, note how long you were using the diet or weight loss method.

In the fourth column, how much weight you lost. In the last column write 'yes' if you ended up in the diet-binge cycle, 'no' if you did not.

*Don't "should" on yourself*
*- Anon.*

## Your Dieting History:

| Name of Diet or Weight Loss Method | Age | How Long On Diet | Weight Lost | Diet-Binge Cycle? |
|---|---|---|---|---|
| | | | | |

## Lesson 4: Breaking the Diet-Binge Cycle

*"I would never have thought I'd be able to get back to eating something without those feelings (guilt and deprivation). I no longer feel trapped. It's amazing not to have thoughts about food and dieting."*
-KR, client

Getting out of the diet-binge cycle is essential to your wellbeing and to managing your weight long-term. You can get out of the cycle at any time, at any point in the cycle. Challenging your need to lose weight, your food rules, and how you think about food and eating will keep you out of the diet-binge cycle forever.

## Commentary on Breaking the Diet-Binge Cycle

Many of us in the industrial world suffer from being trapped in the diet-binge cycle. Much of our pain comes from disconnecting from ourselves and our bodies, including our appetite. We lose the child-like trust in our ability to listen and respond appropriately to our body signals. Conscious and unconscious habits (actions), attitudes (thoughts) and emotions prevent us from enjoying freedom around food, eating, weight and shape. Once we let go, there's the possibility of conscious-choice eating - eating that is completely in tune with the greater cosmos. But this will not occur while we are stuck in our heads trying to figure out a way to lose weight. Our minds are very potent forces for staying trapped or for moving into freedom

The cycle can be interrupted anywhere. As a nutrition therapist, I focus on the upper end of the cycle around disrupting food rules and dietary restraint, because if you can succeed in nourishing yourself on a regular basis you will eliminate any *physiological* reasons for overeating. If you are eating regularly and listening to your appetite (this also means eating foods you love that may not be nutritious) and are still overeating or bingeing, then you will have to explore underlying psychological reasons for your behavior.

Keeping food, mood and appetite records are a starting point. Keeping a record of what and how you are eating can be confronting at first but if you can stay objective about it, it will reveal many things. Accurate monitoring will help you see things you were not able to see before. It gives you answers to questions that you may have been asking yourself for years:

- Why am I eating now?
- Why am I over- or under- eating?
- Why do restrictive or overeating episodes happen?
- What are the triggers for over- or under-eating?

Food, mood and appetite records will also help you to see how you change and make progress. Research suggests that people who keep records recover quicker than people who don't. There is one caveat: If you find yourself obsessing about the record keeping in any way, it will not be helpful.

## In Practice
### Maddy

Maddy was a thirty-six year old woman who migrated from England when she married two years ago. Maddy had never eaten normally. Because her mother had an eating disorder of her own, Maddy's intake had been closely monitored and restricted from when she was a toddler. By the time she was school age, Maddy was overeating regularly. She started dieting as an adolescent, which eventually triggered the diet-binge cycle. Maddy started bingeing daily during adolescence. Her highest weight (130 kilograms) was during her early twenties before she started using compulsive exercise to manage her weight. Though her aim was to keep her weight below 55 kg, her lowest weight as an adult had been 60 kg.

Maddy's motivation to change came after getting married. She and her husband planned on having a family and not wanting to pass on her strange cyclical eating patterns and compulsive exercise she sought help. She had been working with a therapist for many months dealing with the underlying problems of neglect and anxiety. She had stopped the compulsive activity, but was distressed about having gained weight and continued in the

## Principle One: Understanding Your Eating

emotional cycle of deprivation and guilt. At that point she was referred to our clinic for help with normalising her eating and weight. She had tried earlier in treatment to eat more regularly and give up her addiction to diet products, including sweeteners, but had found the anxiety too much to handle.

More than a year down the track, with many more tools for managing her anxiety, she dived into normalising her eating with some conviction. In the first week she cleaned out all low fat and diet products, including the artificial sweeteners she loved, from her cupboards and refrigerator. She started eating more regular meals and snacks and included the foods she had listed on her food fears hierarchy. In the second week she started monitoring her appetite. Maddy discovered that she could recognise when she was hungry and full, though she continued to eat to the meal plan we had set up the first week as a safety net. In the third week, her anxiety went through the roof. She told me she cried a lot that week. Especially on the day she realised that she could no longer spend time with friends who had their own eating issues because it was too much of a trigger for her. What got her through was the loving support of her family. Her key issue now is figuring out what her body wants to weigh. She has a couple of reference points: her weight will be somewhere between 60 kg and 130 kg – her previous low and high weights and her reference weight is in the low 60s to high 70 kilogram range. Her drive for thinness and her desire to lose weight is still strong some days. However the roller coaster of recovery may be a shorter ride for Maddy for several reasons: She is willing to get support from both her family and skilled professionals. She has also learnt to let emotions flow through her and how to manage the more difficult emotions in ways that fit with her values. Lastly she is learning to respect and trust the signals her body is sending. Because Maddy continues to work on both the symptoms and cause of her eating disorder she has every chance of fully recovering and normalising her eating and her weight, despite never having experienced that in her life.

## Happetite Training

Exercise Nine:

Use one of the food record templates on the next page (full page versions available in Appendix 2) to keep a record of what you have been eating and drinking and how your intake is related to your thoughts, feelings, appetite levels and other behaviors over the next week. Also, as always in this process, see the record keeping as an experiment. Maybe start with recording one meal or one day a week. Take it slowly and observe. Just observe. Aim to use the positive part of you that you chose in the introductory chapter, page 25-26.

## Principle One: Understanding Your Eating

Understanding your eating (Dieters)　　Date:　　Day:

| Time | Thoughts and feelings before eating | Hunger | Food eaten and fluids | Fullness | Location | Thoughts or feelings after eating |
|---|---|---|---|---|---|---|
| | | | | | | |

Connections made between food, mood and appetite.

Understanding your eating (Dieters)　　Date:　　Day:

| Time | Thoughts and feelings before eating | Hunger | Food eaten and fluids | Fullness | Location | Thoughts or feelings after eating |
|---|---|---|---|---|---|---|
| | | | | | | |

Connections made between food, mood and appetite.

## Happetite Hints: Principle One

**The Eating Continuum is a scale that describes various types of eating from eating disorders, to disordered eating (including restrictive dieting and overeating), to normal and conscious-choice eating. Acceptance of where you are on the continuum is crucial in order to move towards more conscious-choice eating.**

**Understanding the diet-binge cycle is important in being able to move away from non-appetite driven eating and toward finding your happetite.**

**There are two pathways that result from restrictive dieting, both lead to physiological and psychological difficulties:**

*Pathway One: The Diet-Binge Cycle*
Restriction or thinking you should be dieting or losing weight → feeling deprived physically and emotionally → getting trapped in the diet-binge cycle → challenges to metabolic, digestive and hormonal systems and one's psyche.

*Pathway Two: The Starvation Syndrome*
Restriction → leads to muscle wasting and appetite shut-off → the starvation syndrome → challenges to metabolic, digestive and hormonal systems and one's psyche.

**Disrupting food rules and dietary restraint is an important part of recovery.**

# *Principle Two:*
# *Understanding Your Happetite*

 

This principle is about letting go of the addiction to dieting and finding a way to connect with your internally-referenced appetite, your happetite. This is the appetite that you were born with, the appetite that comes naturally. Your appetite is something like the television remote control: you can adjust the volume and channels without understanding how the television itself works. You can respond to *how* hungry you are (volume) and *what* you are hungry for (channel). You do not need to know

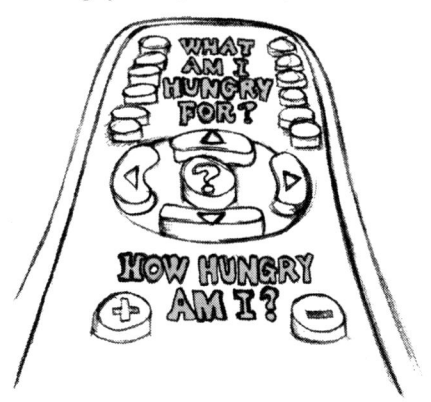

about all the enzymes, hormones and neurological pathways that get triggered when your appetite is engaged, but you do need to pay attention to the signals your body is sending.

If you aren't getting enough food to fuel your body, your ancient brain directs you to find something to eat and puts many of the body systems not required for food-finding on hold until you do. If you go on ignoring your in-built survival systems, you will encounter both physiological and psychological difficulties.

## Lesson 5: DYE-IT (Not Diet) - Ceasing Dieting Behaviours

*"Going on a diet is a lack of self love."*
*- Sarah Magner*

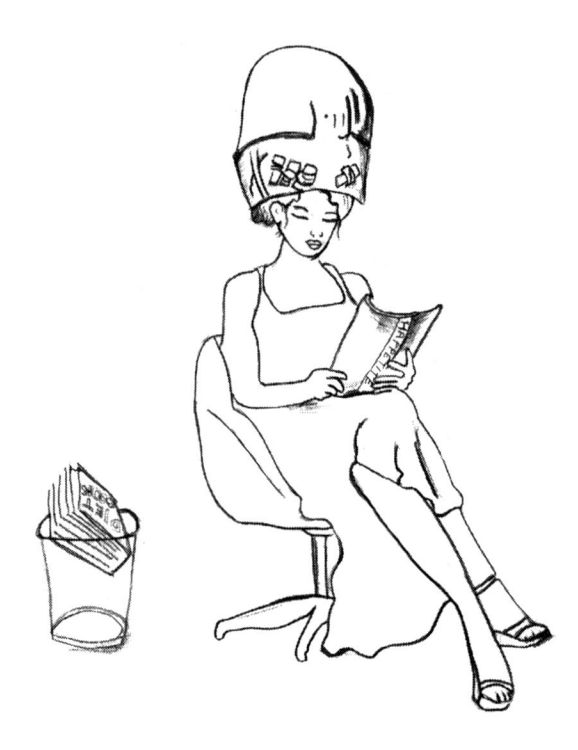

The first step in finding your happetite is ceasing restrictive dieting. The next time you feel fat or overweight, want to lose weight and would like to diet you'd be much better served by changing your hair colour. Buy a bottle of hair dye, or a box of fabric dye, and change the colour of your hair or a t-shirt. It will do more good for your well being than dieting, no matter what your weight or gender. Then ask yourself the question, "What's really going on?"

## Commentary on Ceasing Dieting Behaviours

Yes, avoiding dieting may seem impossible in a food, weight and shape obsessed culture but it is important for your wellbeing that you find a way. Dieting messes with your head and it messes with your body. Even though it does not have a clinical diagnosis, in my experience, restrictive dieting is a form of eating disorder.

Dieting disrupts normal metabolism and digestion crucial to appetite functioning. Dieting leads to low or inadequate intake of vital nutrients like fat and protein, which disrupt brain functioning and are also important for appetite regulation. Somewhere between 60-80% of our brain is made up of phospholipids (lipid equals fat), so fat is necessary in appetite regulation.

Dieting leads to overeating. Always. Whether it takes hours or years depends on the severity of your disconnection from your appetite. The more connected you are to your appetite, the shorter the period of restriction and the sooner you will be overeating. Most likely you will decide to diet again and the never-ending cycle of dieting and overeating (or bingeing) begins. It is a perpetual cycle that makes you feel like there is something wrong with you.

We live in a world that tells us over and over again that we should be dieting. Headlines tell us that we can lose five kilos in two days or that we can look like the latest celebrity by following the latest restrictive diet. However, this sends a message to your body (and your children if you have them) that you cannot trust your body (and your children in turn better not trust theirs). Natural appetite-driven eating, on the other hand, will allow your weight to settle, at a weight your body wants to be and help you trust your body again.

You are able to regulate your appetite perfectly. You always have been able to, you just forgot how. Your mind started making judgments about what is good and bad, how much to eat and how much to weigh.

In a study done in the U.S. in my home state of Iowa, babies were shown to grow consistently no matter how diluted or concentrated the formula was. In other words, they drank more if diluted formula was provided and less if they were fed concentrated formula. Babies are great at self-regulation and so are you, if you can get out of your own way.

The complexities of appetite are described in this excerpt from a science news article:

Hunger, cravings, and satiety are all triggered by a complex network of controls, regulators, feedback mechanisms, and internal signals. Nutrient stores are closely inventoried and signals act on the brain and gut to set off hunger pangs and to drive appetite and eating based on the information – much like a computerized inventory in a store that notifies buyers when stocks are low and new inventory is required.

Dr. W. Sue Ritter is a researcher at Washington State University's Programs in Neuroscience, and it's Center for Reproductive Biology. She studies how the nervous system integrates feeding behaviors, using up nutrients, and maintaining body weight, and how this circuitry strives to achieve a metabolic steady state. One of the main physiological regulators is the level of brain glucose. While the brain requires glucose as its metabolic fuel, it can't store glucose. Because glucose deprivation can be lethal, our brains all have an early warning system that is triggered when blood glucose levels are falling: sensitive detectors fire off powerful nerve, hormonal and behavioral control signals to try to restore normal glucose levels. A number of different hormones [including but not limited to adrenal, corticosterone and glucagon] are secreted triggering increased food intake.

Dr Ritter states: "Detection of glucose deficit activates systems that seemingly or maybe actually commandeer the animal's entire response network. The animal's life is instantly reorganized, priorities are dramatically altered, sensation is redirected, physiology is changed from cells to systems, and reproductive capacity is put on hold. The animal is driven to find and consume food, while its physiology meters out the remaining metabolic fuels."
- *Gray, L. Feeding behavior: studying how the cycles and signals work. [2004] UWHealth Sciences News. University of Washington.*

## Principle Two: Understanding Your Happetite

Eating to your appetite helps give you freedom from weight, food and shape obsessions. For those of you that have been dieting since you were born, the level of fear this statement brings up for you will be an indicator of how important it is for you to begin making changes. The stronger the fear, the more I'd encourage you to feel the fear and do it anyway.

Last year I attended a women's gym over the winter months. One morning I had an interesting conversation with one of the part time workers there. Pip worked as an actress and dancer when she was not working at the gym. She had one of those lithe, toned bodies that other women wish they had. Her mane of dark curls and sparkling eyes suggest she is from the Mediterranean region, though her Australian accent says otherwise. She asked me what I did for a living and when I told her that I work with people who have eating disorders, she in turn told me she had been more interested in nutrition since working at the gym. She noticed that exercise isn't enough for some of the women who want to lose weight. She had been perusing the internet in the hopes of finding a few answers. A drop of sweat fell into my eye as I worked my triceps on the resistance machine. I asked her what she had discovered.

"There is so much information out there – it is hard to sort out what is useful."

She went on to say that her search so far had her leaning in the direction of the Mediterranean-style diet: Tomatoes, olives and olive oil, pasta and fish.

"For some that will work, but what about people intolerant of those foods?" I could hear myself getting up on my soapbox. "Food, cooking and diet books are bestsellers. Why?" I asked Pip the rhetorical question and launched into the answer before she had a chance to reply. "Because the person who wrote the diet book had sorted out the answer to their own food and eating problems with their own specific diet solution and decided to publish it."

Pip told me to relax my shoulders as I pressed into the resistance machine and then continued with the conversation:

"My sister and I were talking the other night and wondering why we are so lucky, both of us are tiny and slim and neither of us has ever dieted." She looked at me earnestly as a shaft of light from the window behind me fell across her high cheekbone.

"Perhaps you are slim because you have never dieted." I suggested.

"We both eat plenty of chocolate," Pip said. She was looking at me as if trying to figure out the conundrum: that eating chocolate could keep you slim.

"It's not the chocolate that is the problem for most people who overeat…"

"It's the portions!" Pip finished the sentence for me.

"Exactly! So it is less about WHAT people eat than HOW MUCH and HOW they eat and HOW they get their other needs met. It's more about their RELATIONSHIP with food. In working with people who have eating disorders I've noticed, all along the continuum of eating, most are out of touch with their appetites. Or if they are aware of their appetite, they don't know how to satisfy it."

In reality the problem is more than just portion-sizes – it is a complex mix of getting our appetites satisfied on a number of different levels. What you are undertaking by finding your happetite is the equivalent of a university course in understanding how you respond to life and figuring out how to separate that from food, weight and eating.

## In Practice
### Jenny

Jenny grew up in an upper class family where dieting and slimness were highly valued. Weight, food and shape were constantly discussed at home and an emphasis on how the women in the family looked overrode all other distinctions.

When first assessed at the Meridian Clinic at Total Heath Care after being referred to us by her doctor, Jenny denied having any concerns about food or weight because it was the norm in her family. In fact, she had a diagnosable case of anorexia nervosa. It took her several months to come to terms with this and many more months of weekly visits to the Meridian Clinic - and a lot of effort on her part - to gain some weight. It was nearly a year before she could start to listen to her appetite. She eventually enrolled in a university interstate and was able to normalise her eating. Once she was out of the family home and could challenge the family conditioning she was able to listen and respond to her appetite.

## Happetite Training

Exercise Ten:
   Begin to take note of how often you have thoughts about:

- Wanting to lose weight;
- Wanting to diet or restrict your food in some way;
- Food in general; and
- Your weight and shape.

   Begin to take note of how often you have feelings of guilt about eating or deprivation about not eating. Jot them down and notice what triggers them. You can use one of the record keeping forms in Appendix 2. The idea is to begin observing what is going on. You aren't trying to change anything just yet.
   For example, when you are craving a food or deciding not to eat something you want, notice what triggered those cravings or thoughts and see if you can make some connections.

Exercise Eleven:
   Go through your kitchen. Clear out any diet foods, diet products and diet books. Note any resistance that might come up around this activity. Be gentle. Do it when you are ready to say goodbye to your old habits. In his brilliant manifesto *In Defense of Food* Michael Pollan recommends "Don't eat anything your great grandmother wouldn't recognise as food." That is great advice - though I'd word it this way: "Aim to eat foods your great grandmother would recognise."

Exercise Twelve:
   The next time you feel fat or overweight, want to lose weight and decide you need to go on a diet, DYE-IT instead. As suggested earlier, buy a bottle of hair dye and change the colour of your hair. Alternatively buy a box of fabric dye and change the colour of something in your world.

Principle Two: Understanding Your Happetite

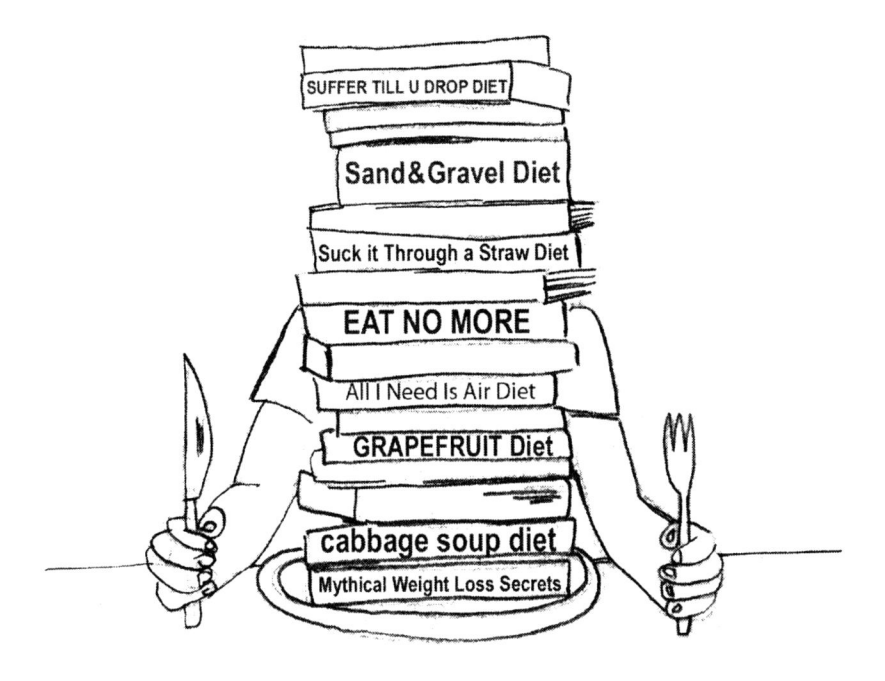

Exercise Thirteen

Repeat exercise twelve each time you think about wanting to lose weight and diet.

## Lesson 6: How Food Rules Affect Our Decisions

The desire for weight loss can trigger the use of restrictive dieting and food rules. Unfortunately, or perhaps fortunately for our survival as a species, there are strong physiological and psychological reasons why food rules won't ever work long term. By being content with your body and your appetite you will be able to listen to your internal cues for hunger and satiety and in turn get to a weight your body wants to be at without using food rules or dieting.

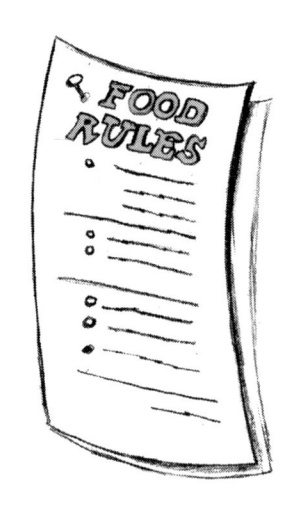

## Commentary on Food Rules Affecting Our Decisions

Dieting and food rules are only a couple of hundred years old. Dieting wasn't even on the agenda until the mid 1800's. (See next page.)

Food rules are intimately linked with eating and weight rules. If you did not think you needed to lose weight you would not be telling yourself not to eat dessert, or that eating after 6:30 p.m. was a bad idea. If your digestive and metabolic systems are working, and you are able to respond to your appetite, your body will be sending appropriate signals to eat or not to eat. Your body will send signals regularly – no matter what the time.

Food rules show up as a judgment about how, what, when, where and why you eat. They no doubt came about because that 'rule' helped someone manage their weight and someone did some research and proved the theory and now you think you are bad if you do not follow that rule.

An example of this is the Overeaters Anonymous (OA) principles. Based on the twelve-step programs of AA, the main goal of OA is to cease compulsive overeating. That is a brilliant goal and one way that might be interpreted is to find a way to return to appetite-driven eating. But in practice, all kinds of food rules are implemented under the guise of the OA principles. For example: avoiding all "white" processed foods. Now there's a food rule!

> **A very short history of dieting (no wonder we're so confused):**
>
> 1829    American Presbyterian Minister Sylvester Graham developed the graham cracker as a way to improve his health. He promoted the use of unsifted and coarsely ground wheat flour for its high fiber content. The flour was nicknamed "graham flour" after him.
>
> 1862    Dr. William Harvey a noted Fellow of the Royal College of Surgeons and an ear, nose and throat specialist, devised a special diet - essentially the first low carbohydrate diet - for his patient William Banting. A year later Banting published the first edition of his now famous Letter on Corpulence in which he tells of Harvey's diet plan. In Banting's words: "I can confidently state that quantity of diet may safely be left to the natural appetite; and that it is quality only which is essential to abate and cure corpulence."
>
> 1863    Dr. James Caleb Jackson created the first dry breakfast cereal which he called "Granula".
>
> 1897    Dr John Kellogg and his brother Will Keith Kellogg started the Sanitas Food Company to produce their whole grain cereals. Eventually they parted ways and Will established the Kellogg Cereal Company.
>
> Early 1900's
>      Horace Fletcher introduced a no fiber, low-protein intake. Fletcher was an American health-food faddist of the Victorian era who earned the nickname "The Great Masticator". He argued that food should be chewed thirty two times – or, about 100 times per minute – before being swallowed.
>
> 1900    Calories are a turn of the century invention and were discovered in a laboratory by chemist William Atwater.
>
> 1918    The book *Diet and Health* by Dr. Lulu Peters was published and introduced the concept of calorie counting to the public.
>
> 1921    Insulin was discovered for treating people with diabetes, and the diabetic diet was introduced. (Clinical diets can still trigger the diet–binge cycle).
>
> Since the 1920's
>      Restrictive dieting has become more popular and consequently food rules have been affecting our lives more and more. Every diet seems to be named after its' promoter or the place it was developed: Stillman, Atkin, Pritikin, Scarsdale, Cambridge, Beverly Hills, South Beach, The Zone. Each devised with the best of intentions, sometimes allowing weight loss in the short term but usually triggering the misery of the diet-binge cycle for dieters (and generating lots of income for its promoters).

**In Practice**
**Alex**

Alex, a 20-year-old sales assistant, was recovering from an eating disorder (Binge Eating Disorder) and was referred for help with ongoing episodes of binge eating. Alex was dealing with the underlying cause of her eating problems through therapy; however her symptoms had not shifted at all over the preceding six months. Daily bingeing had been reduced to two to three times per week initially but she got stuck there. During our assessment it was evident that the bingeing was still being triggered as a result of a very lengthy list of food and exercise rules. Alex was at a normal BMI and, interestingly, did not identify weight as a driver for her bingeing. Instead the drivers were very specific food rules around being healthy and exercising for fitness. Her rigid pattern of eating and exercising prompted the diet-binge cycle the minute she stepped out of her routine.

Alex's first 'homework' assignment was to write out a list of all her food and exercise rules. Her resistance to the task was very high, and after a couple weeks she had still not written her list. Revealing her list of rules meant that she would have to challenge them and she was not sure she could cope without them. She was eventually able to write the list of rules during one of our sessions – but only after the structure of a meal plan provided her with a sense of security about her eating. It took many months of experimenting to prove the rules no longer helped Alex as much as they used to. With the assistance of her therapist she found other ways of managing the underlying anxiety, too. She became 'friends' with her hunger and fullness simply by observing her appetite levels while eating to the meal plan. She eventually discovered that eating to her appetite was an easy way to manage her weight and ultimately that allowed her to let go of the food and exercise rules.

## Happetite Training

<u>Exercise Fourteen:</u>
Make a list of your food, eating and weight rules:

| **My Food, Eating, Weight and Shape Rules** |
|---|
| Examples: |
| Don't eat after 6 pm |
| My ideal weight is - |
| Don't eat ice cream |
| |
| |
| |
| |
| |
| |
| |
| |
| |
| |
| |
| |
| |
| |
| |
| |
| |
| |
| |

## Lesson 7: Good Food/Bad Food Myths

This lesson ties in with the previous one about food rules. We make judgments about all of the foods we eat, how nutritious or non-nutritious, how good or bad they are for us, rather than listening to the cues our body sends us before, during and after eating.

## Commentary on Good Food/Bad Food Myths

In the columns below, under the headings good foods/bad foods, make a list of all the foods that you identify as good, for whatever reason, and all the foods that you identify as bad.

| Good Foods | Bad Foods |
|---|---|
|  |  |
|  |  |
|  |  |
|  |  |
|  |  |
|  |  |
|  |  |
|  |  |
|  |  |
|  |  |
|  |  |
|  |  |
|  |  |
|  |  |
|  |  |
|  |  |
|  |  |

## Principle Two: Understanding Your Happetite

How do you feel about eating the foods in column one?

Here are some adjectives my clients use:
- Virtuous
- Clean
- Healthy

How do you feel about eating the foods in column two?

Here are some adjectives my clients use:
- Guilt-ridden
- Bad
- Dirty
- Unhealthy

Now cross out the word 'Bad' and replace it with the word 'Recovery'. How are you doing? Does it make you feel excited? Terrified? Frustrated? Angry? What other thoughts or feelings did this little exercise elicit? In reality there are no good foods or bad foods. Once you recover from the shock you might be interested to find that the second column is the list of foods that will help you find freedom around food, eating, weight and shape. Quite a mind-bender isn't it?

This lesson is fundamental to recovery and is basic groundwork for getting rid of the Internal Terrorist residing in your mind, constantly harassing you about food and weight. It is also a basic behavior modification technique called exposure therapy, traditionally used very successfully for people who have fears. You have a fear of eating foods that:
- Will make you fat;
- Prevent you from losing weight or
- Impact you negatively in some other way.

For example, you might fear eating something sugary if you have diabetes because it will increase your blood sugar level. You might fear eating a high cholesterol food because it will increase your risk of having a heart attack. Yes, some of your fears may have come about because of the abundant health research readily available, but has that knowledge helped you stay out of the diet-binge cycle? Probably not. In fact it may have perpetuated the diet-binge cycle because your fears are now validated and they intensify the food rules.

Few areas are as faddish as dietary theory. Yesterday's diet edict is today's falsehood. Every so often years of "scientific truth" will be dispelled or at least confused by new research. The Glycaemic Index (GI) revolution is a classic example. From 1921, when insulin was first discovered, until the 1980's when research on the glycaemic index of foods was first carried out, sugar was entirely taboo in the diabetic diet. Research on glycaemic index has transformed how people with diabetes think about carbohydrates. We now know that in combination with other, more slowly absorbed nutrients including protein, fat and more slowly absorbed carbohydrates (low GI foods) the impact sugar has on blood sugar levels varies widely. Yet the rate of Type 2 Diabetes continues to climb. So there is something the research is still missing. It makes sense to experiment with what works to get you out of the diet-binge cycle – even if at first it seems contrary to what you have been told about nutrition and health.

Research on eating competence supports this assertion and suggests that it is an important component of health and overall wellbeing. For example, research using the Ellyn Satter Eating Competence Model showed that people who have high eating competence are more likely to have healthy body weights, have healthier hearts and other indicators of nutritional health. Competent eaters are normal and natural eaters. They have positive attitudes about eating. They enjoy food. They are confident they will have enough food to eat and they trust their bodies' internal references of hunger and satiety. In short, competent eaters are happy with their eating and their natural weight. They are flexible and comfortable with their eating habits and make it a priority to regularly provide themselves with enjoyable and nourishing food.

## Determining Dislikes

There is a group of dietitians in Australia who work in the treatment of eating disorders. Years ago the group debated the question of how dislikes should be handled when patients with eating disorders were admitted into hospital.

On general hospital wards, dietitians, or dietary aides, typically collect a list of dislikes from patients. The disliked food is excluded from the patient's meal trays in order to help encourage an adequate intake during their admission. This activity was straightforward until eating disordered clients were encountered and each had a long list of dislikes and few foods they would agree to eat.

So what to do? Limit the list.

Hazel Williams, a leading dietitian in Australia in the treatment of eating disorders was the first to trial this idea. It worked so well in helping her clients that the rest of us in Australia have followed her lead and limit the list of dislikes to three. The aim is to identify the foods that were dislikes before any dieting or disordered eating behaviours emerged.

## Vegetarianism

The issue of vegetarianism, or vegan diets, often comes up. Research first conducted by Maureen O'Connor in Australia revealed that very often vegetarianism is part of eating disorder/disordered eating. How can you tell if it is not? If the vegetarianism started well before the concerns about food, weight and shape. I usually give a grace period of about six months – if it is within the six months then likely some food and weight concerns were creeping in already and the vegetarianism was just a delaying tactic by the eating disordered part of you. If you want full recovery, I would highly recommend challenging the food avoidances around consuming animal proteins. Otherwise it is a window of opportunity for 'IT' - the disordered eating - to move back in at the first sign of stress. Again as always, go gently. Forcing the issue just leads to resistance. Once you have freedom around food and are eating normally, you are in a position of choice. Then you can decide whether or not vegetarianism is for you. You will be able to tell it is a conscious choice by your ability to stay out of either pathway: the starvation syndrome or the deprivation and guilt-driven diet-binge cycle.

## In Practice
### Sarah

Sarah is a 17-year old student whose mother brought her in for help with managing her disordered eating. Through discussion of the diet cycle she was able to start challenging most of her food avoidances, except three: lollies, chocolate and ice cream.

For nearly nine months, her eating improved steadily. She was able to eat regular meals and snacks and have a certain level of freedom around her food. She said that she disliked lollies, chocolate and ice cream and preferred not to eat them. But eventually she started bingeing again. Normally overeating episodes or binges will include the foods you have been avoiding, but not for Sarah, she binged on other foods and kept avoiding the lollies, chocolates and ice cream.

She hasn't ever been able to confront her fear around these foods and continues to be seen irregularly in our practice for difficulties with restrictive and overeating phases of her eating. When she can finally admit her avoidance of lollies, chocolate and ice cream is being driven by fear of weight gain and not merely because she dislikes those foods, she will be able to bring herself completely out of the cycle of restraint and bingeing.*

---

* One day several months after this was written, Sarah surprised me by bounding into my office with a huge smile and a spring in her step. Her mother, with a pleased expression on her face, was tagging along not far behind. Sarah told me she'd had a chocolate bar for afternoon tea after our session the previous week. She had also started eating lollies and ice cream, too. She had been eating to her appetite all week and her weight had been maintained through the week. What was the trigger during the previous session? She finally connected with the idea that only by eating freely can one's weight stabilise. She will need some time to consolidate the changes but it looks like full recovery is now a possibility.

**Happetite Training:**

<u>Exercise Fifteen:</u>
Expose yourself. This exercise is about challenging food avoidances. Do you:
- Feel remorse or guilt after eating certain foods?
- Avoid eating certain foods?
- Hate to eat certain foods but used to like them before food, eating, weight and shape concerns plagued your life?
- Get rid of food after you eat it by purging? (Purging = chewing and spitting, using laxatives, vomiting, exercising compulsively to burn calories and lose weight or using any other creative method of getting rid of food and losing weight.)

If so, you will hate this exercise and avoid doing it. That is normal. But it will be important to challenge your resistance and take that stance of curiosity we spoke about earlier.

Make a list of all the foods that fit into the following categories. Get a pencil now and fill in this chart:

| Foods I avoid sometimes, often or always: |
| --- |
| |

| Foods I don't eat, because I think they will make me fat, gain weight or prevent me from losing weight: |
| --- |
| |

| Foods I don't like: |
| --- |
| |

| Foods I purge (spitting and chewing, vomiting, exercising compulsively, using laxatives or diuretics) after eating: |
| --- |
| |

| Foods I avoid eating for some other reason: |
| --- |
| |

## Principle Two: Understanding Your Happetite

Be honest. Get someone (parents or siblings perhaps) to help you remember what you used to eat. You can allow three dislikes - foods that you didn't like to eat before the disordered eating started - and exclude genuine food allergies (foods that cause anaphylaxis). If you list more than three you are not being honest with yourself or you were a fussy eater to begin with and challenging your fussiness may be helpful.

In carrying out your own food challenge the first question to ask is:

What foods did I dislike before I had food, weight or shape concerns?

If you still have more than three foods on your list, there are a couple additional questions to ask yourself:

Did I follow the lead with my parent's food avoidances or disordered eating patterns? Am I willing to challenge these?

Some people may drink low fat milk or skim milk because their mother was a chronic dieter and had her own food and weight issues. Perhaps it is because they have been diagnosed with high cholesterol or there is heart disease in the family and current nutrition science suggests that limiting fats helps prevent heart disease. So let's explore each of these possibilities.

First you may simply be a product of your environment. There is the story of the woman who cut off the end of the ham before she put it in the pan for roasting. She was newly married and her husband was puzzled by her behaviour. He asked her why she cut off the perfectly good portion of ham. "My mother always did it," was her reply. So the husband – who it has to be said liked to be right - rang his mother-in-law and asked her why she cut off the end of the ham and she had the same reply: "My mother always did it." Fortunately, Grandmother was still alive, so the husband, who it has to be said was persistent, rang his wife's grandmother and asked her why she cut off the end of the ham. And Grandmother said, "Because the pot was too small."

Think for a minute about the eating skills you learnt from your parents. Which were helpful and which were hindering to your development of deliberate and conscious-choice eating?

Mothers in particular, have a lot of influence around food and eating. In saying this, I do not want any mother to feel guilty about any habits that have already been passed on or any child to lay blame. Guilt and blame aren't helpful and have no place in recovery. Taking responsibility for where you are at now is what is helpful.

So let's now take a look at the second scenario: high cholesterol. High cholesterol can be caused by a number of factors. Stress from malnutrition is one of them - being underweight can cause your cholesterol to go *up*. Hypothyroidism, pregnancy and post-surgical stress are others. The list goes on. Cholesterol is a sterol, a stress hormone, and becomes elevated when the body is under stress. Of course it also goes up, according to current research, when there is too much saturated fat in the diet causing the cholesterol molecules to become "sticky" and cling to the walls of your arteries.

Normal eating means using whole foods. Normal milk is a whole food. Milk is a relatively low-fat product anyway, so to me it seems a bit silly to take out the fat. The theory was that reducing saturated fat in the diet would help with reducing heart disease. But low fat diets were mostly designed for people who had heart disease: men who were over 50 and who were overweight. When the fat is taken out all sorts of changes take place to the new food that is created. In this case, the fat in milk helps with the absorption of fat-soluble vitamin D, which in turn helps with the absorption of calcium, both important nutrients. And who knows what other synergistic effects it has that modern nutrition science has yet to discover. Secondly have a look at your skim or low fat milk nutrition label. There is undoubtedly a long list of food additives. The point is that manufactured food products are not always what they seem and diet products may not be helping with the present epidemic of eating and weight problems. In fact, I believe there is quite a strong argument for the idea they may be hindering progress. The research in the area of eating competence mentioned earlier highlights this.

Now, complete the worksheet on page 92 and then rewrite each food you've listed in a hierarchy in the form on page 96

## Principle Two: Understanding Your Happetite

– from scariest/most avoided to least scary /least avoided food. Next, starting with the least scary food start challenging yourself. Place a tick behind each food every time you eat it. Do not worry if this seems crazy or an impossible task. As you learn more about yourself and your eating you can come back and revisit this exercise. However, do not think you can recover without challenging your fears. **You will not have freedom around food or be able to listen to your appetite until all foods are emotionally equal.** That means that if you were holding a carrot in one hand and a chocolate bar in the other there would be no emotional attachment to either! The decision about which to eat will be impartial and based on your internal references. The neutral questions you might be asking would be something like:

"Which one am I hungry for?"

"How hungry am I?"

"Which will satisfy me the most right now?"

"How satisfied will I feel after eating?"

"How am I likely to feel (physically) after eating it?"

| Rating 1-10 (1= no fear, 10 = strong fear) | **Food Fears (or Food Avoidances) Hierarchy** Giving each food a ranking or score on a scale of 1-10 at the start will allow you to see your progress as you go through the food challenge. For example, chocolate may be a 10/10 to start but after the third test it has dropped to a much lower number indicating the fear around eating chocolate has decreased. |
|---|---|
|  |  |

Principle Two: Understanding Your Happetite

**Lesson 8: Have You Ever Been A Normal Eater?**

Everyone is born with an ability to listen to their appetite - an innate drive to eat regularly and eat a variety of foods. As we grow older however, other influences take over and many of us disconnect from this natural ability to regulate our appetites. Take a moment to think about how your natural appetite has been helped or hindered. Write down your thoughts here:

_____

_____

_____

_____

_____

How would you describe normal eating?

_____

_____

_____

_____

_____

If you were eating to your natural appetite, how would your eating look and feel?

_____

_____

_____

_____

_____

What does hunger feel like for you? What does satiety or fullness feel like after a meal?

_____

_____

_____

Ellyn Satter, a dietitian and social worker in Madison, Wisconsin describes normal eating this way:

"**Normal eating** is going to the table hungry and eating until you're satisfied. It is being able to choose food you like, eat it and truly get enough of it not just stop eating because you think you should.

**Normal eating** is being able to give some thought to your food selection so you get nutritious food but not being so wary and restrictive that you miss out on enjoyable food.

**Normal eating** is giving yourself permission to eat sometimes because you are sad, happy or bored or just because it feels good.

**Normal eating** is mostly eating three meals a day, four or five, or it can be choosing to munch along the way. It is leaving some cookies on the plate because you know you can have some again tomorrow or it is eating more now because they taste so wonderful.

**Normal eating** is overeating at times, feeling stuffed and uncomfortable, and it can be under eating at times and wishing you had more.

**Normal eating** is trusting your body to make up for your mistakes in eating.

**Normal eating** takes up some of your time and attention, but keeps its place as only one important area of your life. In short, normal eating is flexible. It varies in response to your hunger, your schedule, your proximity to food, and your feelings."

**Commentary on Normal Eating**

Normal eating should be as simple as breathing, but it isn't. Living in the industrialised regions of planet Earth has created huge obstacles for listening to our natural drives, including appetite. Schedules, family tradition, culture, modern living, religious practices, food availability, food manufacturing and health issues all impact our decisions about how, what and when to eat. These issues shift decisions away from internal references such as hunger, satiety and how we generally feel after eating. Another way to put it is: our food and eating decisions get made almost entirely 'from the neck up' rather than 'from the neck down'. Certainly the brain and mind are crucial in appetite regulation. What I am distinguishing is the difference between decisions that are intimately connected with our body and physiology and those that aren't.

How do you find out what normal eating is? Have you ever been a normal eater? What was that like? This can take a bit of detective work and often I find having other family members in the room when exploring what normal eating might have been like for you can be very helpful.

Almost always, as part of the initial assessment or very early in treatment, I spend time looking at the last time someone had an experience of normal eating, a time when they were not thinking about their food, weight or shape. It is always an invaluable aid for the client and for me in helping to establish a nutrition plan for recovery.

Most people are able to remember a time when they did eat according to their natural appetite. Usually it's just before adolescence sets in, when we are innocent and impervious to external and social pressures. Sometimes a client can make it through the difficult adolescent phase and then encounter eating problems with a change in lifestyle.

Ask yourself questions like:
- When was the last time I didn't have any food, eating, weight or shape concerns?
- How old was I when I last ate according to my appetite?
- Where was I living?
- Was I at school or in the work force?
- Who was in my surroundings when I ate meals and snacks?
- Where did I eat?
- What times of the day did I usually eat?
- Were meals and snacks served at regular times through the day?
- What foods did I eat?
- What did I drink?
- What portion sizes did I have?

## In Practice
### Jane
Jane was referred for nutrition education and assessment for her eating concerns. She lived with her husband and 3-year old daughter. Anthropometric data obtained included her height of

## Principle Two: Understanding Your Happetite

154 centimeters and weight of 50.5 kilograms, giving her a BMI of 21 (reference range 20-25). She reported she was currently at her highest weight ever and had a past medical history of anorexia nervosa at age 14 when she was at her lowest weight of 30 kilograms. She reported she was not concerned about her weight and wanted to normalise her eating, even if that meant gaining weight. She had been less focused on her weight since she stopped weighing herself two years prior.

Her eating and weight concerns began at age 12, when she cut red meat out of her diet in response to her mother's chronic dieting. Further restrictions developed until age 14 when her mother took her to a physician for treatment. Jane reported that she gradually gained weight and started menstruating when she was 18. She weighed 40 kilograms by the age of 19, maintaining that weight until seven years ago when she began bingeing at age 22. This coincided with her moving away from the food restrictions encountered at home. She saw a dietitian about a year later but did not find the prescribed meal plan helpful and had not tried anything since.

Recently she had been bingeing about twice a week, usually late in the afternoon or late at night. Typically, the binges consisted of the foods she avoided at other times: sweets and high fat foods. She denied vomiting or other forms of purging and reported incidental activity only. On the days she did not binge, she ate restrictively and avoided fat.

Her food recall over a day suggested that she ate three small meals plus three snacks a day and her food choices consisted mostly of low fat carbohydrates. She reported that she had tried to include more dairy and protein foods. Her fluid intake included four drinks per day from water or juice and five to six cups of black tea a day. She took a multi-vitamin daily but no other supplements.

The educational parts of our sessions focused on the diet-binge cycle, exploring what normal eating was like for her before the age of twelve (yes, it took a bit of detective work), reviewing the guidelines for normal eating, challenging her food fears and eating regularly. Jane liked the idea of being able to eat the foods she normally avoided as part of her daily intake but admitted that she found it difficult and guilt-provoking. She was highly motivated, however, and was at a turning point in her life. She wanted to improve her health and wellbeing and was particularly motivated to recover in order to not pass on her habits to her daughter. Because of her level of motivation it took Jane just a few months to normalise her eating.

*"I'm so glad I saw you. After seeing you, I wasn't stressing about food or worrying about what to eat. I could enjoy food without guilt."*
*-E.G., Client*

**Happetite Training**

Exercise Sixteen:
Start exploring your dieting history. Fill out the forms on the next few pages. Write out three separate eating patterns:
1) Your current eating patterns.
2) Your eating when it was at its most restrictive or excessive (or both).
3) Your eating when you last ate normally (you did not focus on food, weight or shape issues). If you cannot remember a time when you ate normally, don't worry. We'll address that situation later.

Principle Two: Understanding Your Happetite

## Current eating

| What foods have you eaten and what have you had to drink in the past 24 hours?: |||
|---|---|---|
| Time | Food eaten and quantity | Fluid type and amount |
|  |  |  |
|  |  |  |
|  |  |  |
|  |  |  |
|  |  |  |
|  |  |  |
|  |  |  |
|  |  |  |
|  |  |  |
|  |  |  |
|  |  |  |
|  |  |  |
|  |  |  |
|  |  |  |
|  |  |  |
|  |  |  |
|  |  |  |
|  |  |  |
|  |  |  |
|  |  |  |
| How typical was the past 24 hours? |||

## Most restrictive or excessive (or both)

| Think back to a time when your eating was most restrictive or most out-of-control and excessive. |
|---|
| Record what you might have eaten in a typical day: |

| Time | Food eaten and quantity | Fluid type and amount |
|---|---|---|
| | | |

Principle Two: Understanding Your Happetite

## Normal Eating – how you ate prior to having food weight or shape concerns

| Think back to a time when your eating was not influenced by food or weight concerns. ||
|---|---|
| Record what you might have eaten in a typical day. Use the questions on page 100. ||
| Time      Food eaten and quantity | Fluid type and amount |

## Are there any other eating patterns you want to record?

| Name: | | |
|---|---|---|
| Time | Food eaten and quantity | Fluid type and amount |
| | | |
| | | |
| | | |
| | | |
| | | |
| | | |
| | | |
| | | |
| | | |
| | | |
| | | |
| | | |
| | | |
| | | |
| | | |
| | | |
| | | |
| | | |
| | | |
| | | |
| | | |
| | | |
| | | |
| | | |
| | | |
| | | |

## *Happetite Hints: Principle Two*

Your appetite is something like the television remote control: you can adjust the volume and channels without understanding how the television itself works. You can respond to HOW hungry you are (volume) and WHAT you are hungry for (channel). You do not need to know about all the enzymes, hormones and neurological pathways that get triggered when your appetite is engaged, but you do need to pay attention to the signals your body is sending.

Avoiding restrictive dieting may seem impossible in a food, eating, weight and shape obsessed culture. However, finding a way to listen to your natural appetite and cease dieting is important to your well-being because:
- Dieting disrupts normal metabolism and digestion.
- Dieting triggers physiological and psychological survival mechanisms that lead to either the diet-binge cycle or the starvation syndrome.

Challenging food fears and food avoidances is an important part of finding your happetite. You will not have freedom around food or be able to listen to your appetite until all foods are emotionally equal. That means that if a carrot stick and a chocolate bar were both placed in front of you there would be no emotional attachment to either.

Exploring your eating and dieting history and remembering what it was like to eat normally, if you ever have, will assist in your journey of recovery.

# *Principle Three:*
# *Clearing the Physical Challenges*

This chapter focuses on the many physical difficulties that can shut you off from being able to listen to your appetite including: metabolic changes, digestive issues, hormonal imbalances, and other aspects including chemicals and pesticides, food allergies and intolerances and the physiological effects of being in the diet-binge cycle.

If you are wanting to diet to lose weight; or if you are over or under-eating in order to cope with other issues ask yourself the question: What is really going on?

**Some Possible Physical Challenges to Finding Your Happetite:**
- ❏ You get low blood sugar levels when you go too long without eating - causing overeating when you eventually do get around to eating - and you need to eat more regularly;
- ❏ Your thyroid is not working properly and you need some medical care;
- ❏ Your hormones have been driven out of balance by yo-yo dieting, pregnancy or lactation, menopause, excess toxins, pesticides or chemicals and you need some medical intervention;

- ❑ You are out of touch with normal appetite signals (chronic dieting, yo-yo dieting and emotionally-driven eating are some of the reasons you may be disconnected from your body and instinctive appetite responses) and need to reconnect with your body's natural signals;
- ❑ You are a shift worker and your natural hormonal and appetite regulation is disrupted and you may need some medical care;
- ❑ You feel out of physical alignment and your "core" needs strengthening through some physical practice such as yoga or Pilates; or
- ❑ You are physically tired and need a nap, massage or bath.

**Lesson 9: Metabolism Basics: Food Intake and Activity**

This lesson is about getting your body in peak metabolic condition and making sure that the food you are taking in is being used by your body. If your metabolism is not working properly you will be prone to moving away from your natural weight and you will suffer from a lack of physical energy.

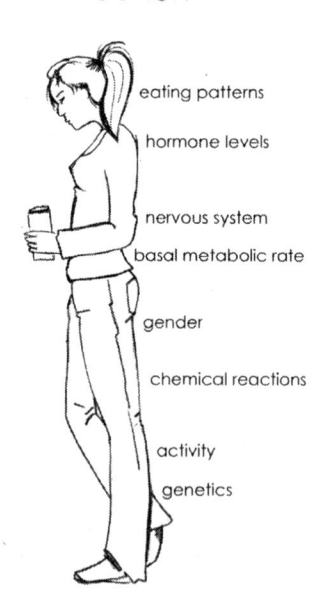

Metabolism is all the biochemical processes that occur within our bodies. It also refers specifically to the breakdown of food and the transformation of food into energy for our bodies. Metabolism also includes the resulting growth, repair, waste elimination, production of energy and cell production. Our metabolism is regulated by our nervous system and chemical messengers composed of hormones like leptin and cholecystokinin (CCK). So, the nervous system and hormones are the stewards of metabolic processes.

**Commentary on Metabolism Basics: Food Intake and Activity**

"What's your metabolic rate?" is like asking how many kilometres per litre of petrol your car gets. Individual metabolic rates may vary enormously, in fact, up to 40% from person to person.

Your total metabolic needs are based on several things:
- Your Basal Metabolic Rate (BMR). BMR is the 'base rate': the fuel needed to breathe, pump blood and keep the automatic processes functioning while you are at rest. This represents 60-80% of the total fuel you use each day.
- The Effect of Activity. The more active you are, the more fuel you will need. There is one exception: if you are restrictively dieting and not meeting your basal metabolic needs the effect of activity can cause you to conserve energy instead of using more – thus slowing down the rate you use fuel. It is an inbuilt protective mechanism to help the survival of our species.
- The Effect of Eating. Nutritionists call this the thermic effect of food. It is the energy needed to digest and metabolise food. Regular eating can increase your metabolic rate, giving you more energy. Breakfast is an especially important meal in triggering how your metabolism functions through the day. Breakfast is a great word: when you eat breakfast you break the fast and stimulate the appetite. The hormones that shut down at night to allow you to get a good night's sleep are reawakened. This is why you may be hungrier and more energetic throughout the day if you eat breakfast. It is also part of the reason why sleep disturbances show up when you are restrictively dieting: your ancient brain sends signals to go in search of food just as our hunter-gatherer

forbearers did during leaner times. BMR varies after meals, but can increase up to 30%. This is why your body is so good at making up for its mistakes when you are eating to appetite.
- Body Size. The bigger and taller you are the more fuel is required for the larger proportion of metabolically active body tissue.
- Age. As you age you generally require less fuel. While your energy needs decrease, your nutrient needs generally increase as you get older.
- Growth. Periods of growth during childhood, adolescence and pregnancy require more fuel.
- Gender. Males have a greater proportion of muscle than females. Muscle is metabolically more active than fatty tissue, therefore people who carry more muscle mass generally have a higher metabolic rate requiring more fuel.
- Infection or illness. Healing and ridding the body of toxins requires extra energy.

All of these affect how fast your body burns up the food you ingest. Dieting slows down metabolism, creating symptoms of starvation whether you think you are starving or not and no matter what your weight.

**A Key Study – Dr Ancel Keys Research on Starvation**

In January 1961, Dr Ancel Keys looked out from the cover of Time Magazine for his contribution to dietary science. Fifteen years earlier, in the northern-hemisphere winter of 1945-46, he was the lead researcher for a government-funded study, now considered a seminal work on starvation and the effects of re-feeding. Re-feeding is a medical term used to describe the introduction of normal eating after a period of starvation. At the University of Minnesota that winter there was a group of 36 conscientious objectors on campus who became more conspicuous as the winter wore on because of their starved and malnourished state. These males had been recruited the previous year for this somewhat unethical experiment, unethical because the

## Principle Three: Clearing the Physical Challenges

researchers asked the participants to starve themselves for six months. It was a humanitarian project in that the research was to inform how to nutritionally rehabilitate prisoners of war. It is a study that has not been repeated for obvious reasons.

The study was divided into three parts:
- The first three months were spent assessing what normal eating was for each participant and recording what the participant's normal intake usually was.
- The second six months involved cutting their intake of food by one half and inducing a state of starvation. The intent was to have each participant lose 25% of their body weight.
- The final part of the study was to determine the best way to re-introduce normal eating.

Here are some of the symptoms Keys and his fellow researchers found during the starvation phase and eventually published in their two-volume, 1500-page report:
- ❏ Depression
- ❏ Apathy (loss of interest in other previously held activities)
- ❏ Irritability
- ❏ Mood swings
- ❏ Poor concentration
- ❏ Dizziness
- ❏ Tiredness
- ❏ Dry skin and brittle nails
- ❏ Slow digestion along with constipation and/or diarrhea
- ❏ Preoccupation with food, weight and shape

Have you ever suffered from any of these symptoms of starvation during attempts to lose weight? Tick the boxes that apply.

Symptoms found during the re-feeding phase:
- ❏ Confusion about hunger and fullness
- ❏ Being hungry all the time
- ❏ Tummy aches and feeling sick

- ❑ Early filling - feeling full before finishing a normal amount of food
- ❑ Rapid weight gain - often experienced for the first week or two of re-feeding. This occurs for a number of reasons, the most significant is usually a result of the body becoming properly hydrated.
- ❑ Night sweats and feeling too hot
- ❑ Spots and pimples on otherwise flawless skin
- ❑ Nightmares and dreams about food
- ❑ Heart palpitations
- ❑ Increased hair loss
- ❑ Uneven distribution of weight gain on the body
- ❑ Poor sleep

Have you ever suffered from any of these symptoms of re-feeding when the pendulum swings to overeating after a period of weight loss? Tick the boxes that apply.

One of the first signals that your body is not getting enough fuel is having constantly cold extremities - the thermostat gets shut down. When you are not getting enough fuel to keep your metabolism firing away, every body system is affected and you will eventually have the following consequences of starvation:

| Body System | Consequences of Starvation | Physical Symptoms |
| --- | --- | --- |
| Endocrine, urinary, reproductive | Thyroid function is depressed, production of the hormone estrogen drops, decreased sex drive | ❑ No menstrual periods<br>❑ No ovulation<br>❑ Vagina becomes dry and vulnerable to infection |
| Skeletal | Calcium loss | ❑ Osteopenia and osteoporosis, loss of height |

## Principle Three: Clearing the Physical Challenges

| Muscle | Muscle wasting | ❏ Looking bony and thin<br>❏ Heart atrophy including possible heart attack |
|---|---|---|
| Skin | Loss of natural lubricants and loss of underlying tissue | ❏ Rough, dry and cracked skin<br>❏ Wrinkles, sags and folds of the flesh |
| Hair and Nails | Protein losses, macro and micro nutrient losses | ❏ Brittle thin and fragile nails, including splitting peeling and cracking<br>❏ Thinning head hair, also losing its shine and falling out<br>❏ Fine downy hair appearing on face, trunk and limbs |
| Mouth | Calcium and vitamin losses | ❏ Reduced saliva<br>❏ Cavities<br>❏ Receding gums resulting in infection and tooth loss |
| Stomach and Intestines | Reduced production of digestive enzymes and reduced | ❏ Food not properly digested or absorbed |

|  |  |  |
|---|---|---|
|  | muscle tone in the stomach and intestines | ❏ Protein deficiency leading to bloating and abdominal distention<br>❏ Sluggish bowels<br>❏ Slow digestion resulting in pain, gas and constipation |
| General | Fluid and mineral losses | ❏ Muscle weakness<br>❏ Abdominal distention<br>❏ Irregular heartbeat |
| General | Metabolic Problems | ❏ Slow pulse<br>❏ Low body temperature (cold hands and feet)<br>❏ Decreased breathing rate<br>❏ Low blood sugar<br>❏ Low blood pressure<br>❏ Low white cell count leading to infection<br>❏ Elevated cholesterol<br>❏ Decreased growth rate in adolescents<br>❏ Water retention |

## Principle Three: Clearing the Physical Challenges

The following chart highlights the physical symptoms associated with refeeding (for the purpose of this book: overeating phases after restrictive dieting):

| Body System | Consequences of Re-feeding (over-eating after dieting) | Physical Symptoms |
| --- | --- | --- |
| Endocrine, urinary, reproductive | Thyroid function may recover, production of the hormone estrogen returns | ❏ Menstrual periods may return<br>❏ Ovulation may return |
| Skeletal | Calcium loss may take time to rebuild. | ❏ Osteopenia and osteoporosis may require further treatment |
| Muscle | | ❏ Heart palpitations |
| Skin | | ❏ Spots and pimples on otherwise flawless skin |
| Hair and Nails | Previous calcium and protein losses, macro and micro nutrient losses take time to replenish | ❏ Splitting, peeling and cracking nails may take time to recover<br>❏ Increased hair loss<br>❏ Hair loss may continue for up to 3 months after re-feeding begins |

| | | |
|---|---|---|
| Mouth | Calcium and vitamin losses take time to replenish | ❑ Receding gums resulting in infection and tooth loss may continue |
| Stomach and Intestines | Inadequate digestive enzymes and reduced muscle tone in the stomach and intestines from previous malnutrition and starvation | ❑ Being hungry all the time<br>❑ Confusion about hunger and fullness<br>❑ Tummy aches and feeling sick<br>❑ Early filling - feeling full before finishing a normal amount of food |
| General | Metabolic Problems – normal metabolic function returns after approximately six months of normal eating. | ❑ Night sweats and feeling too hot<br>❑ Gaining weight unevenly<br>❑ Rapid weight gain initially often due to rehydration |
| General | | ❑ Nightmares and dreams about food<br>❑ Poor sleep |

Because dieting has been such a popular part of our culture for so many years it is hard to think that we do it for no good reason. Dr Ancel Keys' research showed us what happens when diet-induced starvation happens. Another researcher, Dr

## Principle Three: Clearing the Physical Challenges

Ethan Sims, did the opposite. He used normal weight volunteers from a state prison in Vermont and deliberately overfed them until they grew fat. He discovered it was challenging to make people gain weight. Different prisoners needed different amounts of calories to gain weight, but most of them required huge amounts of food in order to gain any amount of weight at all. At the end of the study the prisoners effortlessly returned to their original weights.

### In Practice
#### Tess

Tess was a 20 year-old architecture student when she first came for treatment. She was diagnosed with Anorexia Nervosa and had many of the symptoms of starvation. She was referred by her doctor and, unusually for someone of such a low weight (BMI 15.5), was highly motivated to gain weight and recover. One of the main difficulties for many clients who are underweight is eating a sufficient amount of food for weight gain. Tess was no exception. She hated the overwhelming discomfort of having to feel very full all day long in order to gain weight. She also misjudged portion sizes and, though measuring portions is not recommended long term, she had to measure nearly everything for the first few days. It took her several weeks to start gaining weight even though she added progressively more food to her daily intake. Metabolically her body was 'firing up' as she started to re-nourish herself, the extra fuel was channeled into restoration and repair of her organs and other body systems and there was no leftover fuel for building body tissue. Eventually she was able to eat sufficiently to allow consistent weight gains for recovery. Once she was at the lower end of her target weight range she was able to start normalising her eating and listen to her appetite again.

#### Rebecca

Rebecca had been using overeating as a coping mechanism for most of her life. With a BMI over 30 she was now working to recover from the underlying causes of her overeating which included childhood abuse and neglect. She found it difficult to cope with feeling anything less than very full. Hunger was a completely foreign thing for her. In fact, even the slightest twinge of hunger sent her into a panic. Through keeping food, mood and appetite records for the first few weeks in treatment she gained some trust in the process and eventually agreed to a meal plan to provide some structure. It also provided space in her day to allow unprocessed feelings to come to the surface. The meal plan gave her lots of flexibility and choice – and the structure of three meals and three snacks allowed her to connect to her appetite. The meal plan is always an experiment, never an expectation that it will be followed perfectly but more a tool to help with observing how food is used as a coping mechanism. Over time, Rebecca became less obsessed with needing to lose weight and started working with her counselor using mindfulness techniques. She began doing some physical activity daily. For her it was a combination of swimming, yoga and walking, all activities she enjoyed. She bought clothes that fit properly and made her feel comfortable and beautiful.

It may take some time for Rebecca to fully engage in appetite-driven eating and allow her weight to settle where it wants. In the meantime she is sorting through the underlying causes of her overeating and her quality of life has improved exponentially.

Principle Three: Clearing the Physical Challenges

**Happetite Training**

Experiment Seventeen:
Take notice of your eating over a three-day period. What are the immediate physical effects if you miss a meal or if you overeat? Notice any fatigue, low energy or loss of concentration. Are there any other physical effects you notice?

_____

_____

_____

_____

Exercise Eighteen:
Go back to Your Dieting History worksheet on page 66 – Write an "S" on the worksheet during any of the periods you suffered from the effects of starvation and write an "R" (for refeeding) on the worksheet during any periods of over-eating after restrictive dieting.

Exercise Nineteen:
Go back to the tables on pages 114-118 with the list of physical consequences of starvation and overeating. Tick any of the boxes that apply to your experience, either now or in the past. Do not judge what you find. You are just gathering information.

**Lesson 10: Digestion - Absorption and Malabsorption**
If there is one body system that is fundamental to good health, it is the digestive system. This is the system that converts the plate of pasta you eat one evening into the cells of your body and the fuel for your daily functioning. If you can not digest and absorb what you eat then you will have difficulties maintaining a healthy mind, body and energy levels. The digestive system runs the length of your body from your mouth to your

anus. A proper understanding of how your body's digestive system works can help ensure that everything you eat keeps moving steadily along.

## Commentary on Digestion, Absorption and Malabsorption

Nothing upsets digestion like restrictive dieting. But before we go there, let's review what happens in the digestive tract. Digestion begins in the mouth with the use of saliva and those very handy tools: teeth. Saliva moistens your food so that teeth can then compact it into smaller pieces, ready to travel down the rest of your digestive tract. When you eat enzyme-rich fresh foods and chew your food sufficiently the food enters the stomach laced with digestive enzymes. These enzymes then start the digestion process breaking down as much as 75% of your meal. One of the difficulties with the modern diet is that there aren't enough food enzymes in processed foods. This early digestion process is impacted, making it difficult for your body to adequately digest foods.

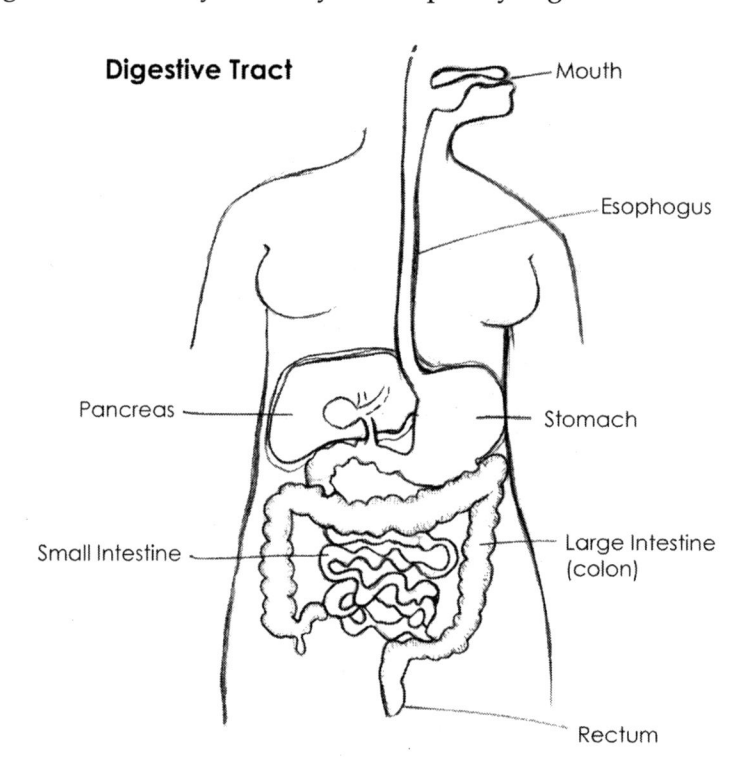

**Digestive Tract**

- Mouth
- Esophogus
- Pancreas
- Stomach
- Small Intestine
- Large Intestine (colon)
- Rectum

## Principle Three: Clearing the Physical Challenges

The stomach is essentially a food warehouse. Empty it holds less than 120 milliliters of solution; swollen with food it can expand up to 30 times to accommodate nearly four litres. Contrary to popular belief your stomach cannot shrink during periods of going without food, but it will feel that way. It is a muscle that stretches much like a balloon: it expands and contracts, continually mixing your food with powerful gastric juices. Hydrochloric acid is introduced in the stomach. The acid inactivates all of the natural food enzymes, but begins its own function of breaking down what is left of the meal. After eating a normal balanced meal it usually takes two to three hours for your stomach to empty itself, signaling to your brain to eat again. That is why it is a good idea during recovery to monitor your appetite after a meal to see how and when hunger shows up again. Fluids and carbohydrates pass through the stomach quickly whereas protein takes a bit longer and fat transits even more slowly, providing the all-important satiety from meal to snack to meal – depending on your schedule and hunger.

Next stop for your food is the small intestine. This is the longest part of your digestive tract. With a normal range of 3 - 7 metres [10-23 feet] long, it snakes its way around itself to fit into your abdomen. Once the nutrient-rich food concentrate moves into the small intestine, the pancreas produces more digestive enzymes to release into the nutrient mix. In the small intestine you finish digesting and break down the meal into the components of proteins, fats, starches and other simpler compounds. Proteins become amino acids, fats breakdown into various types of fatty acids (lipid is another term for fat) and carbohydrates become simple sugars, for example, glucose. Pancreatic juices and bile from the gall bladder help with this process. The presence of tiny finger-like bumps called 'villi' on the inside of the small intestine means that the surface area is much larger than if the lining were just a flat surface. This increased surface area improves the small intestine's ability to absorb nutrients. As the digestive mixture travels through the small intestine, the villi absorb the nutrients and transfer them to the bloodstream and onwards to the liver and muscles. Any food that has not been digested in the small intestine, i.e. fibre (along with some water and vitamins) then reaches the large intestine.

The last food processing stage is your large intestine - the colon. It can take up to 24 hours for the leftovers of the food to push through to its final destination. The job of the large intestine is to absorb any remaining water and store the final product. With some luck, all of the nutrients that you put into your mouth will have been absorbed by the time it reaches the large intestine. Transit time has been positively associated with the amount of digestion, absorption and microbial fermentation occurring in specific regions, or in the whole gut.

> "Movement stimulates healthy and timely elimination. Exercise is like an internal massage for your intestines and colon that helps move waste products along, helping you feel less bloated and more vital. Swimming freestyle requires muscles in the abdomen and torso to work to rotate the body as you slip through the water – and in my opinion it's one of the best exercises to aid elimination. Yoga sequences that include standing postures, backbends, twists and forward bends will also give you a good squish and stretch to keep things moving. In addition to the mechanical benefits, yoga postures increase circulation to the digestive tract, aiding absorption of important nutrients. They also settle our nervous system, literally turning on our 'inner calm' switch, which can be helpful in managing stress, anxiety and the symptoms of Irritable Bowel Syndrome [IBS]*."
> 
> -Felicity Spencer, Physiotherapist
>
> ---
> \* Author's note: Fructose malabsorption is also associated with the symptoms of IBS.

Many people with distorted or disturbed eating patterns experience nutrient malabsorption, in particular because of the lack of enzymes in the gut to help with digestion. In many cases it is insufficient protein or lack of good quality plant foods that is the culprit. Protein is required for the production of enzymes and plants are naturally laden with enzymes. Malabsorption can also occur, in our modern world, due to the ingestion of pesticides and additives to food.

## Happetite Training

<u>Experiment Twenty:</u>
An efficient gut and bowel help you feel great. You can order a complex medical test to see what your transit time is but here is a simpler version you can do at home: Cook up some fresh beetroot and eat them. See how long it takes for the beetroot colour to pass through your intestines and into your stool (yes, you will have to look at your poo). An average transit time can range from 12 to 48 hours. Too slow and you may have constipation and be absorbing toxins you may not want; too fast and your gut will not have time to take up all the nutrients your body needs. Either way, getting off the dieting merry-go-round may be helpful.

<u>Experiment Twenty-One:</u>
Try one of these potential solutions if you suffer from constipation. If these don't get you going then you will need to find out what the underlying cause is (malnutrition, hypothyroidism, pancreatic or gallbladder issues, etc):

1) 2-4 tablespoons of Psyllium husks + a couple extra glasses of fluid each day.

2) Bran – a couple tablespoons on your cereal in the morning along with a couple extra glasses of water during the day.

3) 2-3 dried prunes or a glass of prune juice each day.

4) Legumes – The One Pot Lentil Miracle. See next page. Eating this meal, once a day for 1-3 days is a nearly foolproof way of getting your bowels working again.

5) Replacing gut enzymes – discuss this option with your doctor.

6) Increase gut flora – there are many over the counter remedies. Eating a tub of natural yoghurt with acidophilus, bifidis, casei and other strains of probiotics is a great start. If you need something more potent, have a chat with your doctor, dietitian or naturopath.

If you are taking an iron supplement, talk with your doctor or dietitian about other ways to increase your iron – oral iron supplements can often cause constipation.

# Principle Three: Clearing the Physical Challenges

## The One-Pot Lentil Miracle [serves 1]

In 2004 I attended an Ayurvedic cooking class run by Tim Mitchell at the Intuitive Well – a health and wellness centre in Sydney. Ayurveda is the centuries old Indian way of life that is all about awareness. (Ayurvedic cooking is about cooking with awareness.)

Though some of the words and ingredients may be unfamiliar because they are Ayurvedic, do not let it put you off from experimenting.

This recipe is adapted from Tim's 'Vegetable Subji' and is infinitely variable...the three basic ingredients required for bowel regularity are the oil (or ghee which is clarified butter), lentils and spices, especially the fennel seeds. If you aren't used to using seeds and spices, this is a great introduction. Seeds need to be 'opened' by heating them in the early part of the cooking process and powdered spices are added later. Both seeds and powdered spices store well and add lots of flavour and nutrition to food. Though I've included several optional ingredients, the dish has the most balanced flavours and textures if you include them:

---

**Step 1: Heat in a medium saucepan:**
1-2 tablespoons olive oil or ghee

**Step 2: Add and fry gently until the mustard seeds 'pop' and other seeds are slightly browned and fragrant.**
1 clove garlic, (finely chopped) or a pinch of asafoetida (found in Indian food stores)
1 Tablespoon of fresh ginger, grated
1 teaspoon cumin seeds
½ teaspoon fennel seeds
½ teaspoon mustard seeds or other seeds (optional)

**Step 3: Add lentils and toss through the spiced oil:**
1/3 cup lentils, washed (small puy lentils are ideal, green or brown lentils also work well)

**Step 4: Add liquids; stir well and cook 15-20 minutes until lentils are softening.**
1 cup liquid (stock, coconut milk, or tomatoes, skinned and chopped)

**Step 5: Add vegetables and spice powders and continue cooking over medium heat until lentils are cooked through and vegetables are just softening [usually 10-15 minutes or more, but cooking time will depend on the type of vegetables you use and how finely you chop them].**
1 cup chopped vegetables (Use just one vegetable you love or try a variety if possible – some examples pea, pumpkin and onion, or zucchini and tomato, or potato and spinach, or cauliflower and carrot, Experiment! Use whatever you have in the fridge.)
1 teaspoon of your favourite spice powder (such as coriander or paprika)
½ teaspoon turmeric
Extra stock or water, as needed

**Step 6: Garnish.**
2 Tablespoons sour cream or regular yoghurt (optional – NOT if you use the coconut milk)
2 Tablespoons green herbs - parsley, coriander, basil, etc. (optional)
A squeeze of lemon or lime (optional)

**Step 7: Serve as a meal on its own or with rice and/or salad**

**Lesson 11: Hormonal Influences**

There are enough hormones in the body to make the mind boggle - in fact, not having the right hormones in the right quantity doing the right things, does make the mind boggle, literally. Hormones can have a profound effect on your thinking, mood and of course appetite and weight regulation.

**Commentary on Hormonal Influences**

Since the early 1900s, over 50 human hormones have been identified. In humans most hormones are produced by certain glands called 'endocrine glands'. Hormones control a number of bodily functions including growth, development and reproduction. The word hormone is derived from Greek and means "to set in motion". If your hormones are not doing what they are supposed to, you can definitely feel emotion or conversely a lack of motion, like the train idling at the station with not enough power to take off.

Of the physical blocks that may disrupt your ability to regulate your appetite and weight, getting your hormones properly balanced is one of the most crucial things you can do for yourself. Insulin, thyroid, cortisol and the male and female hormones such as estrogen, progesterone and testosterone all have significant impact on weight and are worth having a chat about with your physician.

Associate Professor Michael Kohn has this to say:

"The importance of these and other hormones that link the bowel and the brain should not be underestimated. More recent evidence suggests that they may also have a role in selecting those who will develop an eating disorder among those who start dieting".

**The Thyroid**

Hypothyroidism - an under active thyroid - is a hormonal problem which can range from mild to severe and can show up at any age, including in newborns. Symptoms can vary widely, which is why it is often missed as a diagnosis. It may produce seemingly paradoxical effects: weight gain or weight loss, fatigue or restlessness, hyperactivity or laziness in children, normal but extended growth leading to taller than average stature or growth failure.

The thyroid is one tiny, but significant organ that is worth getting checked. The thyroid hormones regulate many metabolic processes including growth and the rate at which your body burns up energy. *Hypo*thyroidism means the thyroid gland is sluggish or under active and reduces your metabolic rate. *Hyper*thyroidism means you are in constant overdrive. While there are several diseases of the thyroid, the most common one is Hashimoto's Disease, an inflammation of the thyroid gland that decreases the secretion of thyroid hormones and is an autoimmune disease. Immune system cells that normally defend the body against foreign invaders, such as disease causing bacteria and viruses, attack the thyroid gland instead. About one in every fifteen people in the general population is diagnosed with Hashimoto's Disease. The symptoms include:

- Fatigue
- Feeling the cold
- Constipation
- Swollen face
- Dry coarse skin
- Dry hair prone to breakage and hair loss
- Voice changes such as persistent hoarseness
- Fluid retention (edema)
- Sudden weight gain that cannot be explained by dietary or lifestyle changes
- High blood cholesterol (One study indicated that all patients referred for diagnoses and treatment of high cholesterol should be screened for hypothyroidism as well.)
- Stiff and tender joints, particularly in the hands, feet and knees
- Cognitive changes such as depression or forgetfulness
- Enlargement of the thyroid gland
- In women, heavy menstrual bleeding

Just to confuse things further, sometimes Hashimoto's Disease does not cause any noticeable symptoms. The condition is sometimes discovered during investigations for other, unrelated medical problems.

People with undiagnosed thyroid disorders may have cravings for foods, have a stronger than normal appetite or have difficulty maintaining a natural weight until appropriately treated. Malabsorption has also been associated with thyroid disease. For example, among coeliac patients it has been found that gluten withdrawal can single handedly reverse the thyroid abnormality.

If the addition of thyroid replacement medication is not sufficient to resolve the symptoms of hypothyroidism in a month or two, you may also have adrenal fatigue*, excess estrogen, or a toxic or heavy metal overload which is preventing your body from recovering.

**The Pancreas**

Insulin and insulin resistance, known as Syndrome X or Metabolic Syndrome, also have a huge impact on nutrient absorption and malabsorption, particularly carbohydrate absorption. Insulin is a hormone produced in the pancreas and is needed when food containing carbohydrate is eaten. Once you chew and swallow the food it enters the stomach where the first stages of digestion occur and then empties into the intestine where the food is broken down into glucose molecules. The glucose (the simplest molecule of carbohydrate and another name for sugar) is then carried into the blood stream and all around the body. All the body's cells use the glucose for energy.

In order for that to happen however, the glucose molecules and the body's cells need the help of insulin. Eating food containing sugar or starch is a signal for the pancreas to release insulin into the blood stream. Insulin then acts like a key to move

---

* The adrenal glands produce hormones that help to balance daily ebbs and flows of energy. The adrenals also release hormones when we are under stress – sometimes called the "fight or flight" response. Being consistently under stress may take a toll on the adrenal glands.

the glucose from the blood into the cells of the body. See the diagram below. The more carbohydrate you eat, the more insulin your pancreas releases. If all goes to plan, the cells, fueled by the carbohydrate you just ate, generate energy. This is why marathon runners, who have a need for vast amounts of ready energy, need to eat so many carbohydrate foods.

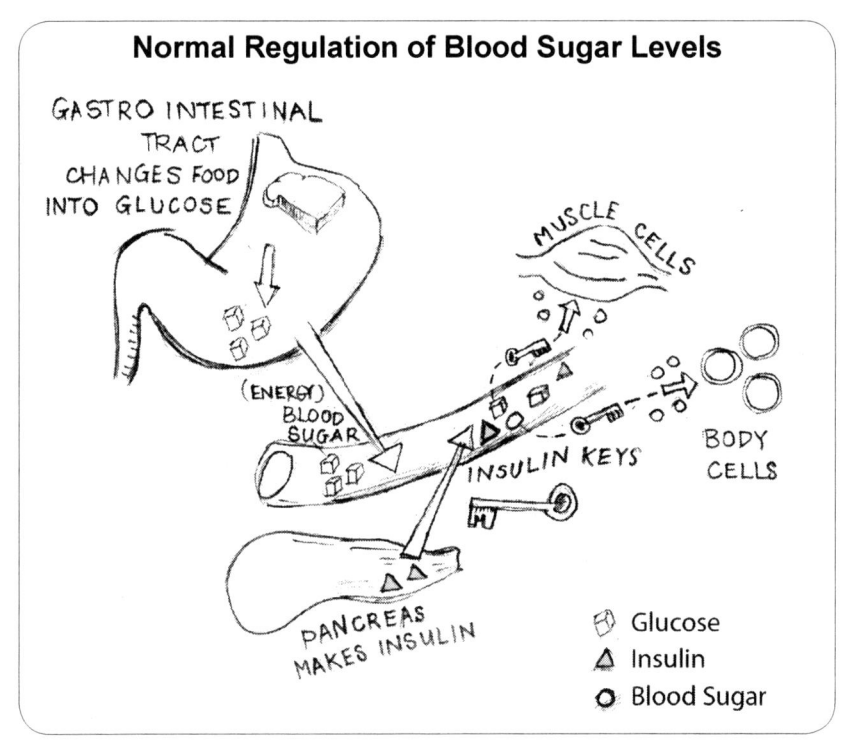

**Normal Regulation of Blood Sugar Levels**

GASTRO INTESTINAL TRACT CHANGES FOOD INTO GLUCOSE

(ENERGY) BLOOD SUGAR

MUSCLE CELLS

INSULIN KEYS

BODY CELLS

PANCREAS MAKES INSULIN

- Glucose
- Insulin
- Blood Sugar

In Type 1 Diabetes Mellitus, previously called early-onset, the pancreas makes little or no insulin. In Type 2 Diabetes Mellitus, previously called adult-onset, though recently more young people are being diagnosed with this type of diabetes, the pancreas may not make enough insulin or the insulin 'keys' may not be working properly. Sometimes excess weight blocks the insulin from moving the glucose in the blood into the body tissues. This is why weight management becomes one of the central principles of managing Type 2 Diabetes Mellitus. It also explains why, with more children being overweight now than ever before, there are also more children diagnosed with Type

2 Diabetes. This is also why many people with this type of diabetes end up in the diet-binge cycle. They are trying to fit into generalised weight management recommendations and following the food rules of the medical practitioners who are in good faith trying to help them.

Symptoms of uncontrolled diabetes include:
- Excessive thirst
- Passing excessive urine
- Tiredness
- Weight loss in some people
- General/genital itching
- Sugar spilling in the urine (identified in urinalysis)

Many people with Type 2 Diabetes Mellitus have no symptoms. Controlling insulin levels and high blood sugar levels is important. While psychologically you may adapt to having high blood sugar levels, your body will suffer the consequences. So it is important to get out of the diet-binge cycle, treat the diabetes and get good control of blood sugars to prevent other complications such as infection, heart and kidney disease, eye problems, nerve damage of the lower limbs and circulation problems.

People with undiagnosed pancreatic disorders resulting in poor insulin regulation (only one part of the pancreas regulates insulin) may have cravings for foods, have a stronger than normal appetite or thirst or have difficulty maintaining a natural weight until appropriately treated.

**Polycystic Ovary Syndrome**

Polycystic Ovary Syndrome (PCOS) is another hormonal problem seen in women. It affects 12-21 percent of women of reproductive age.

Diagnostic Criteria (usually two of these three criteria are required for diagnosis):
- Polycystic ovaries (PCO) are present on ultrasound;
- High levels of male hormones are found in the blood and/or
- Menstrual dysfunction.

Symptoms of PCOS may include:
- Irregular, infrequent or heavy menstrual cycles;
- Weight gain;
- An increase of fat in your upper body;
- Difficulty in becoming pregnant;
- Immature ovarian eggs that do not mature;
- Excessive facial or body hair;
- Acne on both the face and body;
- Prediabetes or diabetes; and
- Higher levels of blood fats.

The way you eat and exercise is as important in managing PCOS as it is in Diabetes. So getting out of any food and diet traps becomes important. Here in Australia, The Jean Hailes Foundation for Women's Health is a gold mine of information and support for PCOS and other hormonal issues. Appendix 3 has contact information for the Jean Hailes Foundation.

**In Practice**
**Jenna (Hypothyroidism)**
Jenna was a 22-year old graduate student who presented to our clinic with Bulimia Nervosa. After several months of treatment she was able to cease vomiting and started on the path to normalise her eating. However, my work colleague, Associate Professor Kohn, came into my office one day saying, "I hope you don't mind, I've agreed with Jenna's plan to follow an 1800 calorie meal plan until she sees you next time." He knows that in order to normalise eating one has to give up the idea of counting calories and thinking about food in such a ritualised manner, but I trusted him and understood there was some reason for him to agree to that.

Jenna soon booked another session and we had a chat about what was going on for her. Despite having challenged all of her food fears and food avoidances, she was still well entrenched into the diet-binge cycle and had resorted to keeping track of her food intake again. In order to prevent her weight from skyrocketing she was limiting her intake to 1800 kilocalories per day. It was all sounding too hard.

Normal appetite regulation (hunger and satiety cues) takes over reasonably quickly once food rules have been challenged and food and weight fears have been eliminated, but this had not been the case with Jenna. I asked Associate Professor Kohn to test her TSH (thyroid stimulating hormone) again. Jenna had an elevated TSH when she first came in for treatment. Sometimes TSH will normalise once the client is re-nourished. However Jenna's TSH was still elevated. She had also discovered there was a family history of hypothyroidism. In retrospect it seemed that Jenna had started the bingeing and purging in response to changes in her weight brought about because of a pre-existing hypothyroid disorder. Because she held strong to a thin ideal, she started to restrict her food intake, which eventually lead to bingeing and finally purging. We referred Jenna to a local endocrinologist - a doctor who specialises in the treatment of hormonal related conditions - to manage her hypothyroidism.

**Dara (Type 1 Diabetes Mellitus)**
Referred by her diabetes educator, Dara was a 29 year-old legal assistant who was diagnosed with Diabetes Mellitus at the age of 19. She'd had the symptoms of Diabetes Mellitus for about three months prior to diagnosis. This was significant as she had been eating very large quantities of food during this time and felt happy about not gaining weight – though because her body's cells weren't getting the fuel she needed she had all the difficulties associated with undiagnosed and untreated diabetes including profound fatigue.

At assessment she weighed 57 kg with a height of 162 cm giving her a BMI of just over 21 (20-25 is the normal reference range). She expressed wanting to maintain her weight, and also wanting to get rid of the bloated feeling she had after eating.

The first time I saw her, Dara was scheduled to have surgery on her feet, which she had injured during kick-boxing. The fractures had never properly healed due to the uncontrolled blood sugar levels she constantly experienced. Dara had recently moved back in with her parents so she would have support during her recovery after surgery.

## Principle Three: Clearing the Physical Challenges

Dara also had a supportive younger sister and a steady boyfriend with whom she spent several nights a week. She described the relationship with her boyfriend as a motivating factor for seeking help. The main motivating factor however, was that she had suffered a diabetic seizure the previous week. She bit her tongue very badly during the seizure and ended up in hospital. She saw this as a wake up call to do something. She described her lifestyle as full of work and drinking. She stated she found health issues neither attractive, nor sexy, and had avoided dealing with them in the past.

Dara described the diagnosis of Diabetes Mellitus as a black cloud that had descended on her. For three months after the diagnosis she did nothing but read about the illness. She dropped out of university and felt depressed. She became exceedingly fearful of diabetic complications, particularly since she had uncontrolled diabetes prior to the diagnosis. She gained weight quickly from 58 kg to 63 kg. Intellectually she knew this was a reasonable weight gain but emotionally she could not cope with it. She started to induce vomiting after meals at age 21. She liked food and found that the all-or-nothing attitude she employed was the only way she could cope. The frequency of vomiting had varied between nothing for a couple of weeks to four times a day, depending on her mood. During our first session she reported vomiting about three times a week and the vomiting was always preceded by a binge. They were ritualistic binges in which she set out all the food beforehand, in the order in which she planned to eat. The binges were relatively small in quantity and apart from ice cream and chips contained mostly healthy or low fat foods that she normally had available in the house, such as rice crackers and vegetables. Her activity included 'pump' classes three times a week for one hour and she did not exercise compulsively.

Though she was eating a couple of times a day, her food choices were very restricted, mostly limited to cereals and grains, fruit, vegetables and other low fat foods. She included some plant proteins occasionally. She prepared meals herself or ate take-away meals.

Helping Dara cease the binge-purge behaviours and normalise her eating were the primary focus of nutrition management plan. She was ambivalent about beginning treatment, but realised she was at a turning point and was motivated to improve her health and well being, in part because of her current relationship and in part because of the recent dramatic diabetic seizure. Her busy lifestyle proved challenging, but eventually Dara, with the help of a therapist and using many of the ideas available in this book, was able to get out of the cycle and normalise her eating.

### Chris (Type 2 Diabetes Mellitus)

Chris had been diagnosed with Type 2 Diabetes fifteen years earlier. Initially she controlled her blood sugar levels through diet alone, but over the past seven years had been taking medication (Metformin) to help increase glucose sensitivity. She had been referred by a diabetes educator at her request as recent ongoing high blood sugar levels had prompted her endocrinologist to prescribe insulin for her. Chris had pleaded her case for more time in the hope of getting her blood sugar levels back under control without the use of insulin.

During our first session she reported having been in a cycle of restraint and overeating for some time, but the fear of having to give herself insulin injections had prompted more severe restriction in the week prior. Though her blood sugar levels were better on the day she was assessed, she was not getting near enough fuel or nutrients for her body. She was also avoiding checking her blood sugar levels, fearing she would have high levels. Our initial session focused on her fear-driven cycle of restraint and overeating. She was highly motivated and was very receptive to the need for detachment and the importance of gathering objective evidence about how her body was working. Education about the diet-binge cycle supported her in setting up a pattern of eating regularly and taking daily walks. She began monitoring her appetite levels and testing her blood sugar levels a few times a day at first and tapering off the frequency of blood sugar testing as she determined through experience what worked and what did not. The effort she put in the first couple of months, including seeing a therapist to help her deal with her fears, was enough to keep her off insulin. Once she accepted that her body *might* have needed insulin she could face what was required for her to get the best possible outcome for her health, whether or not that meant giving herself insulin injections.

## Happetite Training

Experiment Twenty-Two:
Here is a simple home thyroid function test described in *Hypothyroidism: The Unsuspecting Illness* by Broda O. Barnes.

### The Basal Temperature Test
In the morning as soon as you wake up and while you are still laying in bed, test your basal temperature by placing a thermometer under your arm for 10 minutes. People with hypothyroidism often have a low-grade infection (the most common one is sinusitis), so an under the tongue test will measure higher than normal because of the close proximity of the sinuses to the mouth. It is best to check the temperature a few days in a row.

Men – take the temperature any day of the month.

Women (before menarche or after menopause) - take temperature any day of the month.

Women during menarche - take temperature on the second or third day of your menstrual flow.

Normal reading: 97.8-98.2 degrees Fahrenheit or 36.6-36.8 degrees Celsius. If it falls under this range it is likely you have hypothyroidism (or have been stuck in a snow drift for some time). If you are over this range you may have an infection or hyperthyroidism. In either case, it is recommended you have a proper physical assessment and blood test to confirm the diagnosis.

Experiment Twenty-Three:
Have a complete check-up with your doctor. Ask your doctor to check your Thyroid Stimulating Hormone (TSH) and have a random blood glucose test to see what your blood sugar levels (BSL's) are. If you are concerned about other hormone levels also talk with your doctor about that.

## Lesson 12: Taking it Further - Food Allergies and Intolerances

Food allergies and intolerances are common today and increasing in prevalence. Dieting interrupts normal gut function, decreases your metabolic rate and disrupts how nutrients are absorbed, sometimes triggering food intolerances. Sometimes the food intolerances predate the eating problems and may in fact be a catalyst for them. For example, a client with coeliac disease is required to avoid gluten. (Wheat, rye and barley contain gluten along with a host of manufactured food products. Oats can also cause difficulties: though it does not contain gluten it can be contaminated with gluten, for example in food processing plants where other grains are used.) For some the avoidance of gluten brings tremendous relief to their symptoms so their motivation to avoid gluten-containing products is high. For others the impact is more subtle and avoidance of gluten can trigger the diet-binge cycle. Digestive issues such as Irritable Bowel Syndrome - sometimes associated with anxiety issues or high levels of stress – can also be triggers for the development of eating problems. For these reasons proper diagnosis, management and education are essential. Accurate diagnosis of food intolerances usually means several weeks on an 'elimination diet'. It is essential that you communicate any concerns about your eating or food issues with the doctor or dietitian who supervises these protocols.

Food intolerances - very different to anaphylactic food allergies - and other airborne intolerances may also be caused by malnutrition and malabsorption. Additionally there are certain substances that block enzymes from doing their job. Heavy metal toxicity (high levels of copper, mercury or lead in the blood or cells of the body) as discussed in the next section, is often the culprit.

### In Practice
#### Grace
Grace was a 20-year-old medical student with a BMI of 21.4 (reference range BMI 20-25). She had been diagnosed with Irritable

Bowel Syndrome (IBS) at the age of ten and developed Bulimia Nervosa in her late teens. She came from a family where food and weight issues flourished and her mother was perpetually dieting. Both her parents were very health conscious. A therapist whom she had been seeing for some time referred her. Grace had been working with her around issues associated with sexual abuse. Not coincidentally, the abuse had started at the age of nine, a year before the IBS was first diagnosed. This meant that the food intolerances were intricately woven into her world as a compelling coping mechanism and would need to be challenged if she were to ever fully recover.

Grace's normal eating prior to the development of her eating disorder appeared reasonably balanced with three meals and three snacks a day, including a wide variety of food. However, on a deeper inspection of her food and diet history, Grace revealed that her family never had sweets at home. She admitted to binge eating when she went to parties where those foods were available. She described a long and winding medical history with many digestive tests and visits to specialists for constipation, slow digestion and other symptoms of Irritable Bowel Syndrome. Unfortunately, she had been prescribed numerous laxatives and bowel softeners over the years. Her avoided foods list was primarily made up of foods she associated with the IBS and foods she described as unhealthy. We went very slowly at first challenging her ideas about good and bad foods and getting her to experiment with foods she had not eaten in years. Her fear of aggravating her digestive issues meant that many months passed before she could begin to challenge her food fears. Medication was prescribed as support for her anxiety during this time. Unfortunately Grace dropped out of treatment before she could resume appetite-driven eating. Giving up her coping mechanisms was too daunting this time around. Hopefully with ongoing therapy around the abuse, she will eventually be able to motivate herself to challenge her food fears, find other ways to cope and resume normal eating.

## Lesson 13: Taking it Further – Xenoestrogens, Additives and Pesticides

Xenoestrogens are the name for chemicals which, when ingested, behave as estrogens. They include pesticides, petroleum products, plastics and hormones – both prescribed hormones and those found in food, including the antibiotics used in animal feed. The body is always trying to keep everything in balance and these types of substances interrupt that normal balance. The root of the imbalance is estrogen or the chemicals that behave as estrogens. These problems are often clustered together into what is often called estrogen dominance. For example, phytoestrogens mimic the estrogen hormone. Soy products are particularly rich in isoflavone phytoestrogens, which are capable of significantly disrupting human hormonal balance, particularly in men. These problems do not show up on normal blood tests.

Hair tissue mineral analysis (HTMA) can identify heavy metal and toxic overloads which can reveal these sorts of underlying problems. Conventional medicine has historically frowned on HTMA for diagnosis. Inconclusive testing in the first years of HTMA was likely caused by lack of quality control. The literature suggests that is not the case anymore, if a reputable laboratory is used. HTMA is now regarded by many doctors, naturopaths and nutritional therapists as one of the most valuable screening tools available in everyday and preventative health care. My personal experience is that despite normal medical treatment I suffered from symptoms of hypothyroidism until I had a HTMA and was diagnosed with heavy metal toxicity.

There are two ways that things can go wrong in the body when symptoms of heavy metal toxicity arise:

1) There may be a poor intake of nutrients,
                or
2) The nutrients may be blocked from use. This means that though there may be adequate levels of nutrients in a cell, the nutrients are unable to be used. In other words, even if a blood test indicates you have adequate levels of iron you may still have the *symptoms* of iron deficiency.

**Poor intake** may be due to:
1) Lack of nutritious food in the diet;
2) Lack of nutrients in the soil in which the food was grown or
3) Food/produce mismanagement.

**Nutrients blocked** may be due to:
1) Environmental exposure to heavy metals or xenoestrogenic compounds;
2) Metabolic disruption or
3) Digestive incapacity - digestive problems include low stomach acid, lack of digestive enzymes, imbalanced intestinal flora or interaction from medicines.

## In Practice

For many years, despite adequate nutrition, I watched my health deteriorate. I had an ongoing search for help with the chronic and debilitating allergies I'd suffered since I was 2 ½ years of age. (I used to joke that I was a 4-pack a week user. Tissues, that is. The big boxes. Handkerchiefs were insufficient for the amount of mucus my body somehow managed to produce.) I became more exhausted after exercising, more bloated and was chronically constipated despite a diet high in both fibre and fluid. I bruised easily. I had high cholesterol, but because the ratio of good to bad cholesterol was okay none of my doctors ever worried about it – but I knew there was something amiss. My digestion became more and more sensitive and the list of foods I could easily tolerate dwindled, though my appetite was strong. I also had strong cravings for certain foods (peanut butter and dairy foods). I was so incapacitated with food and airborne allergies that I could not get through a day without taking antihistamines. For years I was practically addicted to them. I also suffered from asthma and eczema. I tried everything from traditional medical approaches to the alternative to the downright silly. I became more anxious, slept fitfully, and had a tired body that could not keep up with all the things my active mind wanted to do. I was always intrigued by those who felt invigorated after exercise. I kept myself active but I always needed plenty of

## Principle Three: Clearing the Physical Challenges

recuperative time afterward. I did not feel well: I was constantly suffering viral infections and could not imagine why. 'What is going on?' was my perpetual question. I stayed open to traditional medical approaches and also explored alternative and spiritual avenues. I started meditating and doing yoga but the physical symptoms still plagued me.

It was the emotional stress of dealing with the death of my husband in 2000 that triggered worsening symptoms and eventual diagnostic breakthroughs. Hypothyroidism - finally diagnosed because I asked my doctor to test my TSH - was diagnosed about six months after Andrew died. Though I had suffered from the symptoms of hypothyroidism since adolescence, the severe allergies had been a red herring. Because they were so disruptive to my life, they were the focus of treatment and ultimately a mask for the underlying thyroid and toxicity problems. Once I started on thyroxin, I finally felt some relief from chronic bloating and fluid retention and I lost a couple kilograms because my metabolism revved up. I remained constipated, however, and still felt like I was walking through molasses: I always wanted to go back to bed soon after getting up in the morning. After treatment with thyroxin, I had normal blood levels of thyroid hormone but still had nearly all the symptoms of hypothyroidism. Over the ensuing months, which turned into years, I became frustrated with one doctor after another. All were kind and helpful but no one seemed to really hear me. There was nothing they could do because my TSH levels were normal. I eventually resigned myself to a life of misery. Fortunately I had an ally in my yoga teacher, Kay Crowe. By then I did not have the energy to get through her regular yoga classes, so I started private sessions with her in hope of keeping some form of daily practice. One day I collapsed in a teary heap of exhaustion on the mat. Kay made me promise that day not to give up until I found someone who could help.

It took a year and many visits to other doctors before I found Dr Phil Van Zanden, a general practitioner and environmental physician at the University of New South Wales Health Service. When I met him in November of 2005, 'Dr Phil' did not seem too surprised by the full hand of symptoms I had. He began teaching me about orthomolecular medicine and introduced me to the work of NRS, the Nutrition Review Service, led by Dr Igor Tabrizian in Perth, Western Australia. When I first met Dr. Van Zanden, he had recommended I have a HTMA done. I was skeptical at first. However once he finally convinced me, the results, and the following treatment, proved to be a turning point in my recovery. Copper overload, excess copper in the tissues, was diagnosed. Copper is a mineral essential for health in minute amounts, but it can become problematic when our dietary and environmental exposure is excessive or when various factors interfere with the body's ability to excrete it. Then copper builds up in tissues, interferes with other nutrients - especially zinc which is why I was craving certain foods high in zinc - and wreaks havoc with health, as any heavy metal does. Copper overload, and the resulting zinc disruption, was implicated in every one of the symptoms I had. It is a condition that is quite common, especially among women, because the female hormone estrogen increases copper retention.

Here are some of the other causes of copper overload:
- Exposure to fertiliser and pesticides.
- Use of estrogen medications such as the birth control pill - this is one of the main reasons for the prevalence of copper overload today. Estrogenic compounds are known to increase copper levels in the tissue.
- Slow metabolism - the slower the metabolism of an individual, the more likely he or she is to develop copper overload, regardless of their copper intake.
- Excessive stress or weak adrenal glands - stress dramatically decreases levels of zinc, copper's primary antagonist, and it also weakens adrenal function. Adrenal hormones help stimulate the liver to remove excess copper from the body.
- Exposure to environmental copper - Copper water pipes can leach copper into the water supply if the water is too acidic. In addition, copper compounds may be added to municipal drinking water. They are also often sprayed on produce to prevent fungus and algae growth.

## Principle Three: Clearing the Physical Challenges

- Occupational exposure - plumbers, electricians and petroleum industry workers are at a greater risk of exposure to copper.
- Vegetarianism - Zinc and copper work in a see-saw relationship in the body. Ideally, the two minerals should be in an 8:1 ratio in favor of zinc in the tissues. Plant foods such as soy products, beans, whole grains and nuts all are copper-heavy. When these foods are emphasized in the diet, the all-important zinc-copper ratio can become skewed, leading to the development of copper buildup.

The nutrients and natural hormones that were prescribed as a result of the hair analysis have allowed me to eliminate antihistamines from my life and most weeks I am down to just one box of tissues. My digestion has improved and I have a lot more energy. More than that, I have hope that I can fully recover from the effects of pesticide poisoning, which is what I believe to have caused all the havoc in the first place. It has been a long and winding road. I am not there yet, but with persistence and dedication I am getting there. It turns out all that mucus was helpful. It removed toxins beyond the threshold my body could tolerate, preventing me from developing more serious problems.

I have also discovered that hypothyroidism may be linked to pesticide poisoning and it is possible the increase in hypothyroidism since the 1960s in the Mid-west of the United States, and in cotton growing regions of the world may be related to pesticide use. Not to mention cancers and other more life-threatening problems.

While this section has focused on copper overload there are many other toxins, heavy metals and xenoestrogens that can trigger chronic problems influencing weight and wellbeing. If you are concerned you may have one of these issues have a chat with your doctor or contact an environmental health clinic in your area.

## Happetite Training

Experiment Twenty-four:
If you are interested, have a hair tissue mineral analysis (HTMA). You will need a skilled practitioner to interpret the results.

**In Australia hair analysis can be done through:**
InterClinical Laboratories Pty Ltd (Healthscope)
Unit 6, 10 Bradford Street
Alexandria NSW 2015
PO Box 6467
Alexandria NSW 2015
Phone:     02 9693 2888
Fax:       02 9693 1888
Email:     lab@interclinical.com.au

**In the U.S. hair analysis can be done through:**
Doctor's Data, Inc.
3755 Illinois Avenue
St. Charles, IL 60174-2420
U.S.A
Phone:     800 323 2784 (USA & Canada)
           0871 218 0052 (United Kingdom)
           630 377 8139 (Elsewhere)
Fax:       630 587 7860
E-mail:    inquiries@doctorsdata.com

## Principle Three: Clearing the Physical Challenges

### *Happetite Hints: Principle Three*

There are physical consequences associated with restrictive dieting.

The starvation syndrome and the diet-binge cycle both make appetite regulation difficult, if not impossible.

Metabolic rate is influenced by many things – including how we eat. Restrictive dieting can slow your metabolism and decrease your energy levels.

A strong digestive system, including an efficient gut and bowel, is important for good health and appetite regulation.

Hormones have a profound effect on thinking and mood. They also impact appetite and weight regulation   Changes to one's normal weight can result if hormones aren't in balance.

Food intolerances can be a confounding variable in eating concerns, sometimes restrictive dieting can trigger food intolerances; in other cases food intolerances can be a catalyst for eating problems. In either case appropriate treatment is necessary.

Xenoestrogens are chemicals which, if ingested, behave as estrogens. They include pesticides, petroleum products, plastics and hormones found in some medicines and in food.

# *Principle Four:*
# *Clearing Emotional Barriers*

*"Worry is praying for what you don't want."*
*– Indian Proverb*

Emotionally-driven eating is common. While food is an immediate and easy fix, the impact of eating because you are anxious, angry, sad or happy means that emotions do not get processed properly and the cycle is perpetuated.

Fat is not a feeling. Fat is a condition. You are fat or you aren't. There are people who are thin who feel fat and others who are fat and feel thin.

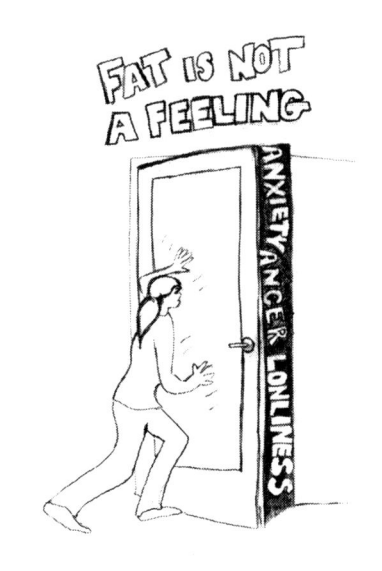

If you *feel* fat then you have to ask yourself: Why do I *feel* fat? What emotion is underneath the *feeling* fat? There will always be one. When you have the thought 'I *feel* fat', pause for a moment and see if you can replace the word 'fat' with an emotion. Some common emotions that trigger feeling fat include worry, anxiety, loneliness, frustration and anger. But the list is ultimately as long as the list of emotions. Which emotions does feeling fat mask for you?

If you *are* fat (BMI greater than 30) then you have to look at a broader picture – in addition to exploring the underlying emotions, you will also have to explore what your weight is about. There are people who eat to their appetite who are overweight or fat. If that describes you and you do not already have body acceptance then that is your challenge. There are also people who were slim once upon a time and are now fat. If that is the case then you will have to explore when and what caused you to start gaining weight and what have been the blocks to appetite-driven eating and achieving a normal weight. In the meantime, can you also be moving towards body acceptance?

If you are feeling fat and wanting to diet or if you are over- or under-eating in order to cope with other issues ask yourself the question, what is really going on?

## Principle Four: Clearing Emotional Barriers

**Here Are Some Possible Emotional Barriers:**
- ❑ You suffer from bouts of anxiety or have an anxiety disorder and need to learn helpful ways of coping.
- ❑ You have an 'unconscious driver' running your life. This might be something like, "I'm really angry my sister was born when I was three and I'll never get over that!" or "I was an only child and I'll never get over that." Unconscious drivers are irrational to our conscious mind. They don't make sense and they produce habits that don't make sense.
- ❑ You operate your life out of a negative core belief, e.g. "I'm worthless" or "I'm undeserving" or "I'm unlovable". You will need help from a therapist that can support you in releasing these unhelpful beliefs.
- ❑ You are angry at your partner/mother/father/sibling/friend for (fill in the blank) and need to express that in a way that moves your life forward.
- ❑ You are feeling sadness or grief and need to cry or release those feelings in a healthy way.
- ❑ You are feeling lost and need some direction (consulting your Global Positioning System usually won't help in these situations).
- ❑ You are feeling confused and need some clarity.
- ❑ You are feeling misunderstood and need some empathy.
- ❑ You are feeling trapped and need some spontaneity/freedom/release.
- ❑ You are feeling ugly and need some self-care and acceptance.
- ❑ You are feeling bored and need to identify what emotions are underlying the boredom.
- ❑ You are stressed and need more balance in your life.
- ❑ You may fear feeling hunger or fullness and you will have to learn how to listen to and trust your appetite again.

**Lesson 14: Psychological Effects of Dieting**

When I first started working in the field of eating disorders, I did not understand the significant impact of proper nourishment on one's mood. I would often send clients back to the psychologist in an attempt to get them to deal with the underlying issues first. It took some time before I understood that re-feeding and nourishing the body and mind were essential in taking care of the psychological issues. Adequate nutrition and regular meals are important mood regulators.

**Commentary on Psychological Effects of Dieting**

Have you noticed you get moody when you are restrictively dieting? These are some of the psychological symptoms that show up from under-eating according to Dr Ancel Keys' research:

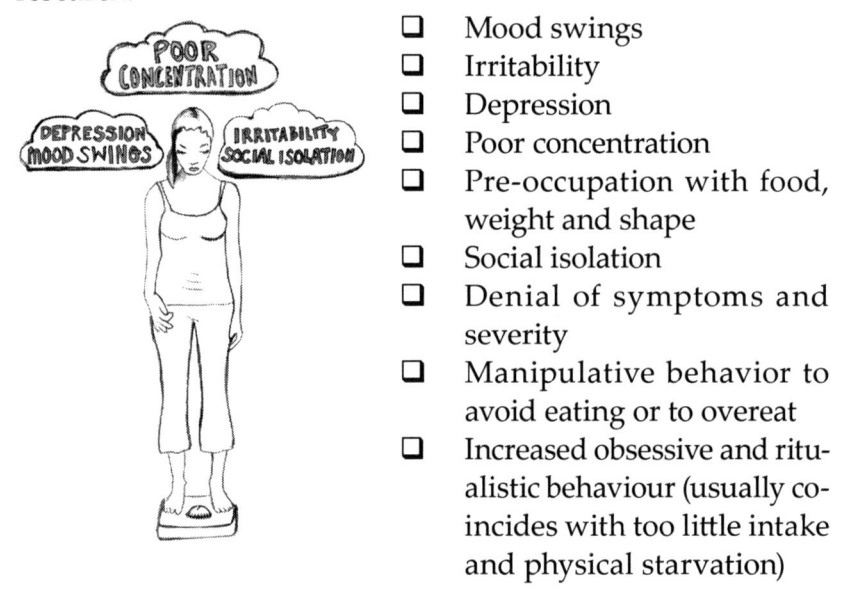

- Mood swings
- Irritability
- Depression
- Poor concentration
- Pre-occupation with food, weight and shape
- Social isolation
- Denial of symptoms and severity
- Manipulative behavior to avoid eating or to overeat
- Increased obsessive and ritualistic behaviour (usually coincides with too little intake and physical starvation)

We are affected physically and psychologically when we are not getting enough food to fuel our brain. We literally cannot be ourselves. Depression and low mood have become commonplace in modern culture, nearly as common as restrictive dieting. I wonder if there is a correlation.

## Principle Four: Clearing Emotional Barriers

Hilde Bruch, in her seminal works on anorexia nervosa, discussed the effects of malnutrition and noted that they masked some of the underlying psychological deficits and recommended re-feeding first before doing any other therapy.

Paradoxically, when we are eating too much - and this can mean too many calories and not enough nutrition - many of the same symptoms show up. What to do? Let your appetite be your guide.

## In Practice
### Kate

Kate is a 53-year-old banking administrator. She remarried two years ago after an acrimonious divorce and has custody of a teenage son from the previous marriage. Her parents are ageing and requiring more attention and she is also now step-parent to an autistic child. Diagnosed with depression a year ago, she has been prescribed medication. Having gained 20 kilograms in the four years since her divorce, she was referred to our clinic by her doctor for weight reduction. During our first session Kate acknowledged she had no motivation to lose weight and could barely get through the day with all her other responsibilities. She felt trapped because if she didn't do something now she would likely only gain further weight. She felt the medication had increased her appetite, but that it had also helped manage her low mood, again a feeling of being stuck. Her eating patterns were largely driven by family and work schedules. Often missing meals early in the day, she had started a pattern of binge eating after work. It was easy to see how much pressure Kate was under from every corner of her life and apart from her doctor and husband she had little support. Previously her mother had been a capable helper but last year had been diagnosed with early dementia and the tables had started to turn. Kate was now the helper to her mother. The session was spent exploring Kate's ability to take time out for herself and get support. She was open to accessing support services through her corporate human resources department and asking her husband and her brother for help. One of the side effects of her medication was an increase in appetite so the doctor tapered her off that antidepressant and started another. She started keeping food and mood records and over time was able to eat regular meals and snacks through the day. Because she was more nourished physically and psychologically; she was eventually able to normalise her eating and get back to the weight she had easily maintained prior to the divorce.

**Happetite Training**

<u>Exercise Twenty-Five:</u>
Have you noticed mood changes when you are over or undereating? Which psychological symptoms have you experienced related to your eating? Tick any that apply and then identify the top three:
- ☐ Mood swings
- ☐ Irritability
- ☐ Depression
- ☐ Poor concentration
- ☐ Preoccupation with food, weight and shape
- ☐ Social isolation
- ☐ Denial of symptoms and severity
- ☐ Manipulative behavior to avoid eating or to overeat
- ☐ Increased obsessive and ritualistic behaviour (often coincides with too little intake and physical starvation)

Are there any other psychological effects you have noticed?
- ☐ _____
- ☐ _____
- ☐ _____
- ☐ _____
- ☐ _____
- ☐ _____
- ☐ _____

**Lesson 15: Acceptance of Weight and Appetite**

Remember what you were like as a kid, think back to a time where you felt free in your body. Maybe lying in bed after a busy day or as a kid swimming in a sagging faded swimsuit and not caring. Perhaps it was eating a mouth-watering wedge of watermelon in the summer with juices running down your face, or standing in awe of nature by taking in the sights, smells and sounds of a spring rain. Think of a moment when weight and shape wasn't an issue and food only brought pleasure: how it looked, smelled, tasted, felt on your tongue; before, during and after eating. What might it feel like to have that experience again? This is your possibility.

**Commentary on Acceptance of Weight and Appetite**

Children have an innate ability to live in the moment. They may have a short attention span but their focus and ability to engage with the natural world is awe inspiring. As we mature, external forces that impact our life in myriad ways often distract us. Lack of time, money and other sources of stress prompt us to start living outside the moment and worrying about the future or fretting about what happened yesterday. We start to use ways of coping that impact how we eat and care for our body. We disconnect from our appetite and ourselves. And perhaps we model that to our children or it affects the way we care for them.

Stephanie Dowrick, a Sydney therapist and newspaper columnist highlighted this in an article in a weekend news magazine:

"Perhaps we expect such (emotional) literacy to be natural, and never more so than in the relationship between parents and their children. Yet quite plainly this is not always the case. A few days ago I sat near the front of a bus taking me into the city, a journey of about 15 minutes. During that time a well-meaning mother shoveled an entire glass jar of food into her plump one-year-old son, despite his eloquent protests. He pursed his lips, screwed up his nose, shook his head, whimpered and turned his head away, and each time he opened his mouth to protest more loudly, she put the spoon in.

As if that were not enough, the mother talked at him constantly telling him how tasty the food was and how much he was enjoying it. Her reality totally obliterated his. In fact, his signals remained incomprehensible to her. I am assuming this was not because she is a bad mother. She is probably devoted to her son, but still she could neither read nor interpret his needs as being in any way distinct from her own

agenda….As this child learns that his signals mean so little to his mother, he will also learn to distrust his own inner signals and instincts, around food, emotions and connections of many kinds. His capacity to read himself will be suppressed or become confused."
– 'Reading the Signals' from Inner life by Stephanie Dowrick in Good Weekend, Sydney Morning Herald, 9 May 2009.

## In Practice
### Jackie

Jackie is a 35 year-old accountant in a de facto relationship with a personal trainer. At the time we met she was training regularly for sporting events such as short runs and triathlons. Jackie was initially referred to us by her physician, for concerns about her compulsive activity leading to recurrent muscle injuries. Jackie had a BMI of 18 and was still dissatisfied with how she looked and performed. She was training more but doing worse at events. She was putting more and more pressure on herself to eat healthier and improve her fitness. Her partner was also putting similar pressure on her.

Her eating had been entirely normal until her childhood sweetheart broke up with her ten years earlier at the age of 25. She went through a six-month period of stress-induced food restriction, but because of the positive feedback she got from the people around her, she determined to keep her weight low. She started running every morning as a way of managing her weight. She entered sporting events on a regular basis as a way to keep herself motivated and that is how she met her current partner. Eventually however her restricted eating and compulsive exercise prompted a malnourished state causing osteopenia, a condition where bone mineral density is lower than normal. It is considered by many doctors to be a precursor to osteoporosis. She began suffering from serious muscle sprains and injuries. When she first presented to the Meridian Clinic at Total Health Care she was hoping to get information to help gain back her competition readiness. She struggled to come to terms with the notion that her body needed time to recover and that she would need to regain weight back to her normal weight. She began seeing a therapist and started dealing with the underlying grief of the breakup ten years earlier. She re-examined her current relationship and set limits so that she no longer felt pressured to perform in competitions. She struggled with the anxiety that came up when she abstained from all but the gentlest of activities. Her mother was diagnosed with a life threatening illness during this time and she relapsed into restrictive eating. Jackie noticed how quickly her energy levels and overall health deteriorated and that motivated her to work harder towards recovery. She attended the clinic intermittently for several years, gradually gaining back her weight, health and stamina. She relearned how to trust her appetite. The last time we saw her she was at a normal weight. She had started competing in triathlons again, this time for the sheer joy and pleasure she experienced. Jackie was pleased with how well she was doing, in the competitions and in life.

Principle Four: Clearing Emotional Barriers

**Happetite Training**

Exercise Twenty-Six:
Think back to the time when you last ate normally, when you didn't have any concerns about food, weight and shape. Write down when that was.
- ❏ Where were you living?
- ❏ What were you doing at that time in your life?
- ❏ Were you at school?
- ❏ Who was living in your household?

Now describe in detail what that was like for you. What was your experience with food, eating, weight and shape? If you have never eaten normally according to your appetite: what do you imagine that might be like?

_____

_____

_____

_____

_____

Exercise Twenty-Seven:
Review the normal intake you wrote down in Principle Two page 105. Is there anything you wish to add to what you wrote?

_____

Exercise Twenty-Eight:
Imagine what it would be like for you to go back to eating like that for one day. What emotions does it bring up for you? Just observe using the positive part you chose back in the introduction.

How do you feel? (Tick all those that apply.):
- ❏ Excitement
- ❏ Relief
- ❏ Fear
- ❏ Trust
- ❏ Mistrust
- ❏ Belief
- ❏ Disbelief
- ❏ Anger
- ❏ Joy

Remember you are still just gathering information. Be observant.

**Lesson 16: The Potion: Emotion**

> *"I realized I didn't have a problem with food –*
> *I had a problem with anxiety."*
> *-N.B., client*

When we pay attention to our emotions we move mountains. In order to progress along the continuum to conscious-choice eating, one of the fundamental steps, if you are an emotional eater, is developing emotional intelligence. By that I mean being able to identify, accept and honour the emotions that well up in you. When you have access to your emotions you also gain access to your appetite, for food and other needs. In turn, during this journey of self-discovery, you will learn to acknowledge your needs and learn how to meet them. Your emotions will always help you find out what your needs are.

> *"Emotional intelligence is the innate potential to feel, use, communicate, recognize, remember, describe, identify, learn from, manage, understand and explain emotions."*
> *- S. Hein, 2007*

## Principle Four: Clearing Emotional Barriers

**Commentary on The Potion: Emotion**

Much illness can be attributed to unreleased and unprocessed emotions, which get trapped in the body, sometimes known as emotional armouring. The countless 'negative' things that happen during our lives can actually benefit us by raising our perceptual awareness and perhaps creating unusual sensitivities. By processing the feelings that did not get processed when we were younger, whether the processing is conscious through psychotherapy or unconscious through bodywork or other therapeutic processes, those childhood happenings can work for us and not against us. As humans we tend to blame ourselves for what happened to us as children: we internalise it as 'I wasn't good enough' or 'I wasn't lovable enough'. But we are not responsible for what happened to us as children, we are however, responsible for our own healing process.

Just as there are as many ways of normal eating as there are people on the planet; there are as many ways of identifying and releasing emotional pain. What have you found helpful?

Below are a few ideas to experiment with.

**Meditation**

Meditation is a powerful, safe and simple way to release emotional blocks that impact eating issues. As a bonus it also positively impacts physical and mental states. There are two basic types of meditation: focusing or mindfulness. The focusing types of meditation use the principle that placing one's attention on something (the breath, an image, or a sound/mantra), helps to still the mind and allow a greater awareness and clarity to emerge. Examples of focusing meditations are Vedic meditation (or Transcendental Meditation) which uses a mantra, and Vipassana meditation which uses the breath.

Laboratory studies of practitioners of Maharishi Mahesh Yogi's Transcendental Meditation (TM), carried out by Benson and Wallace at Harvard Medical School towards the end of the 1960s, provided the first detailed knowledge of the many physiological changes that go with meditation. The physiological changes were different in many ways from those found in sleeping people or those in hypnotic trances. Meditation produces 'a complex of responses that marks a highly relaxed state'. Moreover, the pattern of changes they observed in meditators suggested an integrated response, mediated by the central nervous system.

In mindfulness meditation the principle is to sit quietly and witness whatever goes through the mind, not reacting or becoming involved with thoughts, memories, worries, or images. This helps to gain a more calm, clear, and non-reactive state of mind.

**The Sedona Method**™*

Another brilliant, subtle and immediate tool for emotional release is The Sedona Method. The work of Lester Levenson and Hale Dwoskin is summarised beautifully and succinctly in the book, *The Sedona Method: Your Key to Lasting Happiness, Success, Peace and Emotional Well-being*. In his introduction to the book Dwoskin states:

"We live in a world that's in a state of rapid change and not all of it is positive. Most of us crave a certainty, security and solidity that we cannot find outside of ourselves no matter how hard we try, but these qualities already exist within each of us waiting to be revealed. It is as though we possess an inner wishing well or a fountain of joy and vitality that's disconnected from the water supply. Yet, secretly, everyone has a tool to reconnect".

The Sedona Method is genius in its utter simplicity and immediacy:
**Step 1:** Focus on an issue you would like to feel better about and allow yourself to feel whatever you are feeling.
**Step 2:** Ask yourself one of the following three questions:
Could I let this feeling go?
Could I allow this feeling to be here?
Could I welcome this feeling?
**Step 3:** Then ask yourself the simple question: Would I? In other words: Am I willing to let it go?

---

* Information used with the permission of Sedona Training Associates.

**Step 4:** Ask yourself the simple question: When?
**Step 5:** Repeat the four steps as often as needed until you are free of that particular feeling.

**Naming and Acknowledging Feelings as They Surface**

If you have difficulty identifying feelings here is a list to help you get started:

| Apathy | Grief | Fear | Anger | Acceptance |
|---|---|---|---|---|
| Courageousness | Lust | Abandoned | Pride | Happy |
| Peace | Guilt | Anxious | Rejected | Serene |
| Obsessed | Shame | Regret | Annoyed | Decisive |
| Fixated | Frantic | Envious | Aggressive | Confident |
| Depressed | Hateful | Greedy | Righteous | Creative |
| Sad | Disgusted | Impatient | Cowardly | Focused |
| Lonely | Unloved | Frustrated | Doubtful | Powerful |
| Worthless | Worried | Hostile | Failure | Spontaneous |
| Lost | Embarrassed | Outraged | Hurt | Optimistic |

The website www.the-emotions.com has a list of emotions and their definitions. You can also go to www.eqi.org/fw.htm for what is purported to be the world's longest list of emotion words that describe feelings.

Your emotions will tell you how you are doing in getting your needs met. Whether you feel happy, sad, hurt, angry, joyous or grateful, your emotions are like traffic signs advising of a bump in the road or a traffic light providing signals about how to proceed. If you are not getting your needs met, you will find coping mechanisms, like eating or not eating, to help you survive until you figure out how to get those needs met.

Sometimes feelings are held in the unconscious. If you find yourself numbing out and losing track of your feelings, the help of a psychologist or therapist is recommended.

## 'Grounding' Activities

Grounding activities get you in touch with your body and can help with the release of emotional and muscular 'armouring'. Gardening or certain types of dancing, such as Kundalini dancing, or body work such as massage and acupuncture will help move the emotions through your body system so that you are freed from their effect on your eating and food choices.

Felicity Spencer, the physiotherapist who works with our team at the Meridian Clinic at Total Health Care, recommends mindful movement practices such as yoga and tai chi, not only for conditioning the physical body, but also as a way to become more at peace with your emotions:

"Active meditation practices like yoga and tai chi keep us tuned to the present moment through movement and breath, while guiding us to greet emotions as they arise. From this point our challenge is not to place these emotions at the centre of our awareness, nor push them away, but to let them float in the background as we gently direct our attention back to the body. Through this we learn how to pay attention to our physical and emotional selves in an open, accepting and nurturing way. This is a challenge, but offers a great reward: the ability to find, even amidst chaos, a sense of peace and wholeness."

## In Practice
### Haley

Haley was an adolescent referred to us by a psychiatrist who was treating her for anxiety and Obsessive Compulsive Disorder (OCD). Her mother accompanied her to the sessions. Haley had obsessive and rigid patterns of eating to cope with underlying anxiety. She ate exactly the same foods from day to day. The pattern had become so restrictive over the previous six months that not only had she stopped growing, she had also lost weight during a time when adolescents would normally be gaining 4 or 5 kg. She lived with the fear that if she changed the types of food she ate, she would gain weight.

Haley felt hunger but would not respond to it. Obsessive compulsive behaviour and restricting her food were her main coping skills. She had recently spent some time in hospital to help her overcome some of her food fears and to give her family a break. She was also initially prescribed medication* to help with the underlying anxiety. She loathed meal times, as did her family because of the conflicts, measuring of food and fear of weight gain. She could not eat away from home because of her unrelenting need to wash her hands.

Treatment started by having her challenge simple things like having jelly, instead of rice pudding, white bread instead of grain bread and replacing a caffeinated soft drink with one without caffeine. All foods were 10 out of 10 on the fear food hierarchy, except for the foods eaten daily.

Through the course of treatment Haley regained some weight and started to manage her anxiety and that allowed some movement in her eating behaviours: she started being more flexible. It was a big milestone when she was able to eat at a friend's home for the first time in five years.

Haley now likes to eat and looks forward to meals, eating nearly everything her mum serves. She is coping with anxiety without using obsessive compulsive behaviour and food restrictions as often, but still struggles with both symptoms and cause.

---

\* Medication can sometimes be helpful in the early stages of treatment. Like a leg cast and crutches can sometimes be helpful when a leg is broken, the medication helps while the brain heals and new coping mechanisms are developed. You should always discuss the pros and cons of using medication with your doctor.

**Happetite Training**

Experiment Twenty-Nine:
Explore one or more ways that you can start to release emotions. Four were discussed in this chapter: meditation, the Sedona Method, naming and acknowledging feelings as they surface and the use of grounding activities. What else might you try or what else has helped in the past that you could experiment with again?

Principle Four: Clearing Emotional Barriers

Exercise Thirty:

Create your 'Joy List'. Make a list of all the things that give you joy. By noticing what gives you joy and aiming to find time for those things in your life, some of the more negative emotions automatically become displaced. The caveat here is to ensure that the joy you are feeling is just that, joy. Not an escape that creates a biochemical high such as a process addiction (compulsive eating fits into this category along with gambling, shopping and obsessive devotion to religion or work as other examples) or substance addiction like alcohol, drug or tobacco abuse. If you do find that these processes or substances are giving you a short-lived high with consequences to your life and relationships then please have the courage to seek treatment. These issues often coincide with disordered eating/eating disorders and full recovery cannot happen without dealing with the addictive behaviours.

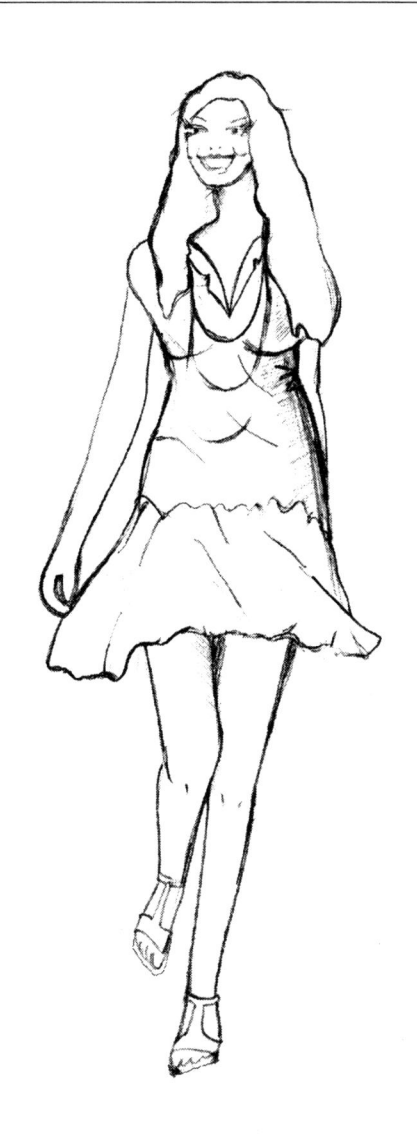

### The Joy List

I created my first 'Joy List' in 2002 when I was doing some personal development work with Alicia Power. Alicia now calls herself a soul mentor and helps her clients tap into their highest, heartfelt desires. At the time, I was on a teleconference call with several others and Alicia asked us to write down what gave us heart-felt joy. I filled two pages itemizing the simplest of pleasures such as swimming in the sea, meditating, listening to music or having coffee with friends. I also included travelling and personal development. Not one of the items generated money or involved what I called 'work'. I resolved during that phone call to fill my life with more joyous moments. Within a year I had reduced my workload and made sure that everyday involved several items from my 'Joy List'.

Exercise Thirty-One:

Start a gratitude journal. Here is what Sarah Ban Breathnach, author of *Simple Abundance*, a book I highly recommend, says:

"There are several tools that I'm going to suggest you use as you begin your inner exploration. While all of them will help you become happier and more content and will nurture your creativity, this first tool could change the quality of your life beyond belief: it's what I call a daily gratitude journal. I have a beautiful blank book and each night before I go to bed, I write down five things that I can be grateful about that day. Some days my list will be filled with amazing things, most day just simple joys."

## *Happetite Hints: Principle Four*

Fat is not a feeling, it is a condition; there are always emotions submerged underneath the 'feeling' fat.

An ability to identify, accept and honour the emotions that well up in you is part of recovery. It releases the emotional blocks that prevent you from listening to your appetite.

Sometimes feelings are held in the unconscious. If you find yourself numbing out and losing track of your feelings, the help of a psychologist or therapist is recommended.

Several ways of identifying and releasing emotions were explored in this chapter. Which ones resonated with you? Which ones are you willing to experiment with? Are there others you have heard about that you are willing to explore?

# *Principle Five:*
# *Motivating Yourself for Change*

*"All creative scientists know that the true laboratory is the mind, where behind illusions they uncover the laws of truth."*
-*Jagadis Chandra Bose*
(quoted in 'Autobiography of a Yogi' by Paramahansa Yogananda)

If you are feeling fat and wanting to diet or if you are over or under-eating in order to cope with other issues, ask yourself the question, what is really going on?

**Here Are Some Possible Mental Blocks to Listening to Your Happetite (These Will Lower Your Motivation to Change.):**
- ❏ You have been a yo-yo dieter and are trapped in the diet-binge cycle. You may feel there is something wrong with you. You need help from someone familiar with the diet cycle; someone that can help you move away from your habitual patterns. (The diet-binge cycle has mental, physical and emotional aspects to it.)
- ❏ You are mentally tired and need a walk, some fresh air, a nap or a chat with a friend.
- ❏ You have all-or-nothing or black-and-white thinking and need to see where you are making progress.

❑ You are in a cycle of negativity and need to be grateful for what you do have.

**Lesson 17: Getting Ready**

Mind your mind. Your thinking is a very powerful tool in recovery from food, eating, weight and shape issues. What are the reasons you picked up this book? What are the reasons you want freedom around food and eating? What do you want for yourself and your life? What do you need to do to get what you want? How can you stay focused on what is working? Having a readiness and willingness to make change is a very important component of finding your happetite.

**Commentary on Getting Ready**

In his 1994 book *Changing for Good*, psychologist James Prochaska and his colleagues identified that people who succeed at making permanent, positive changes, go through identifiable stages of change. The five stages he identified are:
- Pre-contemplative
- Contemplative
- Preparation
- Action
- Consolidation

There is an ebb and flow between the stages of change, in other words it is not a linear process. Honouring where you are at in the stages of change will help move you forward. This is a key principle in making changes to your life around food, eating, weight and shape. Here is a summary of each stage.

**Pre-contemplation**

Pre-contemplation is summed up in the statement, 'I don't have a problem'. When you are in pre-contemplation you may be getting feedback from others that you have a problem but you are not yet ready to acknowledge that a problem exists. Other ways the pre-contemplation stage presents itself is that you become defensive when the problem is mentioned and refuse to

### Principle Five: Motivating Yourself for Change

talk about it or you think your problem is "hopeless" and cannot be solved. Pre-contemplation always comes with resistance to change.

**Contemplation**

If you understand there is a problem but have not yet made a decision to change then you are contemplating change. Contemplating change can produce fear and anxiety. The thought of giving up what is familiar and/or having to develop a "new self" can be paralysing. Avoiding or postponing change is easier. However, there is also curiosity about what benefits there may be in giving up the problems – you start to weigh up the pros and cons of your current situation.

**Preparation**

During this stage, you are actively planning for change. You have set a goal for yourself and will be able to make statements along the lines of: "I want to stop dieting; I want to trust my appetite again. I will start to normalise my eating by working towards having breakfast every day."

**Action**

This is the stage of change where you do it – where you begin to eat regularly, start exploring how your appetite works, and begin trusting your body. Perhaps it is one meal at a time at first, but building gradually to eat regularly through the day, every day. This is the stage where you start to remove the physical, mental and emotional blocks to listening to your appetite; where you begin to substitute positive behaviours for unhealthy ones and helpful thoughts replace limiting thoughts and beliefs.

**Consolidation or Maintenance**

This is the long-term process that keeps you experimenting until slips or lapses are no longer a concern. Maintenance helps guard against a return to unhelpful and unwanted behaviours. Slips are to be expected as a part of recovery. You start seeing slip-ups as a time of greater learning against the backdrop of the smaller distinctions you make when things are going smoothly. You may notice you often learn more from your slips ups than you do when things are going well. You learn to persevere during the course of recovery and do not get discouraged by setbacks.

Recovery from an eating problem is a passage through these stages. Understanding why you want freedom around food, weight and shape will help keep you motivated during the roller-coaster ride that is the process of change.

**Rolling with Resistance**

Rolling with resistance is a very useful tool during any of the stages of change. It means noticing how you defend your position and "rolling with" your excuses for lack of change. All resistance is a form of fear. Fear arises when we encounter situations that we think we cannot handle. Many fears arise during our childhood when we are powerless – and then we carry those fears with us into adulthood.

Helen Storey, a Sydney-based nutrition expert in the treatment of eating disorders, often relates the fear and trepidation (the resistance) of crossing a moving, flexible suspension bridge over a raging river as a metaphor for the journey of recovery. Tentative steps, shaky footing and holding on for dear life are all part of the crossing. As one lets go of the fear and rolls with the movements of the bridge the journey becomes easier, even enjoyable. The adventure of the crossing opens us up to other possibilities on the other side of the river. And so it is with recovery.

Recently I participated in the resistance and fear-inducing experience of firewalking, a centuries old initiation rite of passage for many cultures. It entails walking across hot coals. Kurek Ashley was our firewalk leader. Having taken thousands of people across the coals safely, Kurek is a top fire-walk instructor and also holds the world record for the longest fire walk. During the training he helped us connect with the power of our focus. He taught our group that we have unlimited potential and can do whatever we want when we are focused and take action. The firewalking is merely a metaphor for harnessing that personal power.

## Principle Five: Motivating Yourself for Change

As each person stood at the head of the line, confronted with the lane of searing hot coals, their resistance and fear became palpable. Kurek 'rolled with' each person's resistance and helped them move into a place where movement was possible. Never forced, each person was, with Kurek's guidance and expertise, eventually able to walk across the coals.

> "If you can walk on hot coals and not burn your feet, your mind must have a powerful influence over your body. Firewalking is a wonderful example of the mind-body connection at work, and a means of demonstrating that we do have control over the process. Over the years a number of skeptics have come up with various theories about why firewalkers don't get burned, but the fact is that some people do get burned while others don't."
> -Adams, C. *Can You Walk on Hot Coals in Bare Feet and Not Get Burned?*

Janey, one of the other participants had this to say afterwards, "I started in fear, moved into power and walked into ecstasy - the transformation was amazing". Here is the equation:

Fear → Power = Ecstasy

During the pre-contemplation stage, rolling with resistance allows you to create an environment for contemplating change. It does not mean condoning your thoughts, feelings or actions but by noticing, and not reacting, you move into the arena of the non-judgmental observer. Some people call this the 'neutral mind'. Others call it the 'wise mind'. By using your neutral or wise mind you can figure out what motivates you to stay where you are. There are always very compelling reasons for doing what you are doing.

After that, you can move on to contemplating what might motivate you to try something different. Then you have the possibility of walking through your fears into ecstasy. The idea here is to focus on what is working and do more of that.

Prochaska's research, along with others, has been developed into a modality of therapy called Motivational Enhancement Therapy (MET). Motivational enhancement research has identified that there are four themes crucial in engaging reluctant clients (or the resistance in yourself):

1. The use of psycho-educational material – material that helps you understand why you do what you do. *Find Your Happetite* is an example of psycho-educational material.
2. Examining the advantages and disadvantages of the symptoms.
3. Using experimental strategies.
4. Exploring personal values.

The idea behind motivational enhancement is to work with someone (or yourself!) in a collaborative way with openness, curiosity, patience, focus and systematic inquiry and allowing individual discovery. Have a look at that last sentence again. What would you need to do to take that sort of stance with yourself?

**In Practice**
**Marni**
Marni is a 29-year-old woman who has suffered from Anorexia Nervosa for 14 years, nearly half her life. She has been contemplating change for some time and alternates between the pre-contemplation, contemplation and action stages of change. She told me that she should be happy when she owns her own home, has regular work and the financial means to do whatever she wants, but she is trapped in sadness, hopelessness and frequent suicidal thoughts . The only thing that gives her some relief is her eating disorder. She imagines the eating disorder as her only true friend, the only thing that can assuage her dark emotions. But the pain of these emotions has been superseded by the pain of the eating disorder. She continues to struggle with accepting and acknowledging all the emotions associated with past trauma. While she works with a therapist on those issues and gets some support from medication, our sessions are aimed at providing a 'voice of reason' against the Internal Terrorist's voice that says she does not deserve to eat or be at a natural weight. A healthy, normal weight for her will be at the upper end of the reference BMI range and about 10 kg above her current weight. She has good weeks and bad weeks while she contemplates the sweeping changes

that are necessary in order to recover. Gradually she is learning that the structure of the meal plan and maintaining a certain minimum weight gives her some space for thinking about longer-term change.

## Happetite Training:

Learning about and training in MET has greatly changed how I work with clients. The following are some of the tools used in the various stages of change in the symptom management of eating problems. Try experimenting with the ones that coincide with the stage of change you find yourself in.

Note: Most people wanting to learn to listen to their appetite have been experimenting with recovery for sometime. Once they reach a point where they have to start trusting themselves and their bodies again they can cycle back into the pre-contemplative stage for a while. Always remember that recovery is a process and wherever you are at is fine.

<u>Exercise Thirty-One: Enhancing Motivation</u>
**Experiments to Try If You Are In the Pre-Contemplation Stage:**
Ask yourself open-ended questions beginning with how, why and what. For example: How is this behaviour helping me? What are the triggers for my binge behaviours? Why am I choosing not to eat?

Ask yourself why others are concerned about your dieting or other behaviours. For example: Why are others so concerned about my compulsive exercise?

Become more informed about the behaviour others are telling you to change. Ask yourself why you have not identified your compulsive actions as a problem.

Try to discuss the problem with someone with whom you feel safe.

Ask yourself whether or not you are behaving in a potentially dangerous way. If so, are there steps you can take to keep yourself from harm?

**Experiments to Try If You Are In the Contemplation Stage:**
One of the most helpful tools to use at this stage is to develop a list of pros and cons for staying with your current behaviour and for change. It can be very helpful to have someone with an objective viewpoint work on this task with you.

## Principle Five: Motivating Yourself for Change

The chart will look like this:

| Benefits of current behaviour | Drawbacks of current behaviour |
|---|---|
| | |
| Benefits of change or recovery | Drawbacks of change or recovery |
| | |

Keep a journal. Notice and write about your moods and emotions.

Get angry at the eating disorder/disordered eating for how it interferes with your life. Read books or watch movies that will inspire you. Picture yourself a year, five years, ten years from now, with the problem and then without it.

Notice how your thinking helps or hinders you from moving forward. Notice how your thinking can trap you: all-or-nothing thinking, waiting for the magical moment, wishful thinking or negative thinking.

When you are ready, set a goal that is achievable and maintainable. Behavioural goals are specific and achievable. For example:

I will eat dinner with the family two nights this week.

or

I will set up an appointment with the doctor by next Friday.

When it comes to normalising your eating and weight, it is important that goals are achievable. As always, use the experimental process.

**Experiments to Try If You Are In the Preparation Stage:**

Go public with your goal and find support - friends, a therapist, etc.

Find ways to set up your environment that will promote success.

You will also need alternative coping strategies - what works in one situation may not work in another.

Have a list of rewards and reinforcements for doing the experiments, whether or not they move you forward. Just doing the experiment is an achievement. The rewards can be verbal or tangible, small or large but ideally they will be immediate.

Having a plan to help cope with inevitable slip-ups is also important.

**Experiments to Try If You Are In the Action Stage:**

Structure your environment. You will find some tips in Principle Seven.

Extend and expand your support structure: friends, doctor, dietitian, etc.

Make a list of nurturing activities to use during times of stress. For example taking a bath, getting a massage, painting, writing in a journal or calling someone you trust.

Use support.

Avoid places that may trigger unwanted behaviour.

Reward successes, even the small ones.

Use distraction when old habits present themselves.

**Experiments To Try If You Are In the Maintenance Stage:**

Be watchful for environments, situations, unexpected stress and a false sense of security that can trigger urges to return to old behaviours.

Support your plan for action.

Reward successes, even the small ones.

Evaluate your action plan regularly and keep the focus on what is working.

## Lesson 18: The Problem With Freedom

With freedom comes responsibility. Freedom around food and weight issues will open you up to other possibilities, but it also means saying good-bye to some dearly held beliefs. Being free of food, weight and shape concerns means you have to take responsibility for your life, your eating, and your response to physical, psychological and mental triggers.

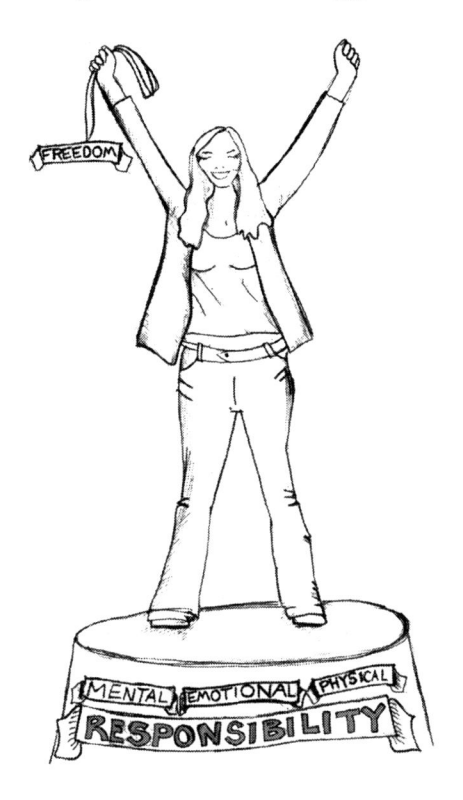

In my work, as part of a medical team, we practice from a treatment model which uses the results of research, evidence-based practices and good old clinical observation. The keyword in this sentence is practice. Any professional is still practicing, gaining and learning from experience and ongoing research. We are practising...and we are practising on you! So, while a professional may be an expert in their area it is very important for you to take responsibility for your part on the team. You are the expert on YOU.

**Commentary on the Problem With Freedom**

Part of the reason thinner people tend to stay thin is that they do not want to lose weight. They already match the cultural ideal so have no desire to go up against their natural physiology. Those of us who do not fit the cultural ideal - or think we don't fit the cultural ideal because plenty of studies show that a big percentage of the population desires weight loss even though they are at a normal weight - start mistrusting our body and our natural physiology. The research I conducted on body image twenty years ago when I was in graduate school, suggested that the image of ourselves as adolescents is the one we carry into adulthood and that is still borne out today. Therefore it seems important to view our body image as just that, an image or mental construct, and work to challenge any negativity we carry around regarding how we see ourselves.

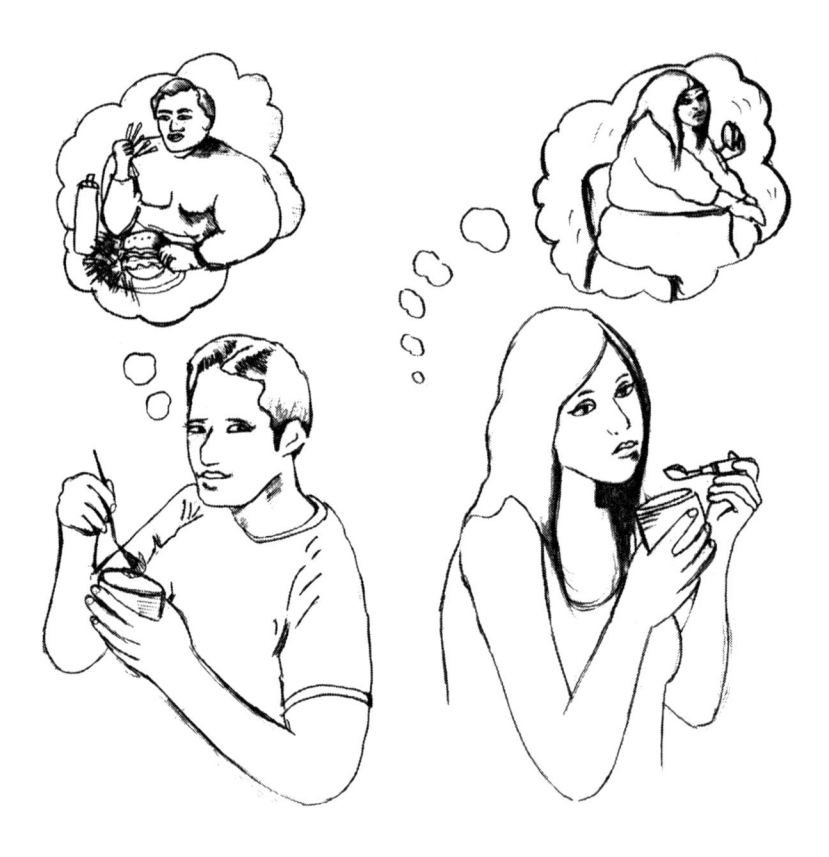

## Principle Five: Motivating Yourself for Change

We start thinking we need to lose weight and then the struggle begins: restriction, deprivation, overeating, guilt. Our physiological mechanisms (digestion, metabolism, hormonal balance and cellular structure) start working towards self-preservation by disrupting normal healthy functioning. We become entrapped. We want freedom from the prison of food and weight-related concerns but the challenge then is to figure out a way to deal with:

- Emotions that we may not wish to experience;
- Emotions we may not even be aware of;
- Our negative thinking;
- Being at a weight other than our fantasy weight;
- Taking responsibility for our health and wellbeing; and
- The idea that we deserve to eat well and nourish ourselves.

**Happetite Training**
<u>Exercise Thirty-Two:</u>
Take an honest appraisal of your situation. Complete the following statements:

I am already taking responsibility for my health, weight and wellbeing by:

_____

_____

_____

However, I still feel unable to take responsibility in these areas of my life:

_____

_____

_____

Because:

_____

_____

_____

I, _____, am now willing to take more responsibility for how I respond to physical, emotional and mental triggers. Taking personal responsibility in these areas may help me recover.

## Principle Five: Motivating Yourself for Change

Physical issues I may be willing to investigate in order to recover include:

_____

_____

_____

_____

_____

Emotional difficulties I might consider exploring in order to recover include:

_____

_____

_____

_____

_____

Thoughts and beliefs I might consider challenging in order to recover include:

_____

_____

_____

_____

_____

**Lesson 19: Externalising the Problem**

Michael White, a visionary social worker and family therapist from Adelaide, South Australia, was the originator of the narrative therapy approach. Two particularly significant principles used in this approach to therapy are maintaining a stance of curiosity and asking questions to which you genuinely do not know the answers.

Another concept taken from the narrative approach which has been picked up and used successfully in eating problems is 'externalisation' of the problem. Externalising the problem, even naming it, helps with the process of observation and making change.

**Commentary on Externalizing the Problem**

A variation of this concept was introduced in the first chapter with the idea that there are different parts of ourselves and the request to notice and use the ones that would help us on a journey of discovery. This process of externalisation is articulated beautifully in the book *Life Without Ed* by Jenni Schaeffer and Thom Rutledge. In the book, Jenni describes her relationship with Ed (Eating Disorder), and how she eventually divorces 'him' in order to find herself and regain control of her life.

See diagram on the next page for an example of a Venn diagram showing this concept of externalisation. Identify how much of the day is spent under the 'cloud' of negative thoughts and behaviours relating to food, weight and shape as you commence treatment and check back regularly to see how you are progressing. The Venn diagram is very useful in assessing progress as you move through recovery.

## Self and Disordered Eating Behaviour – Venn diagram

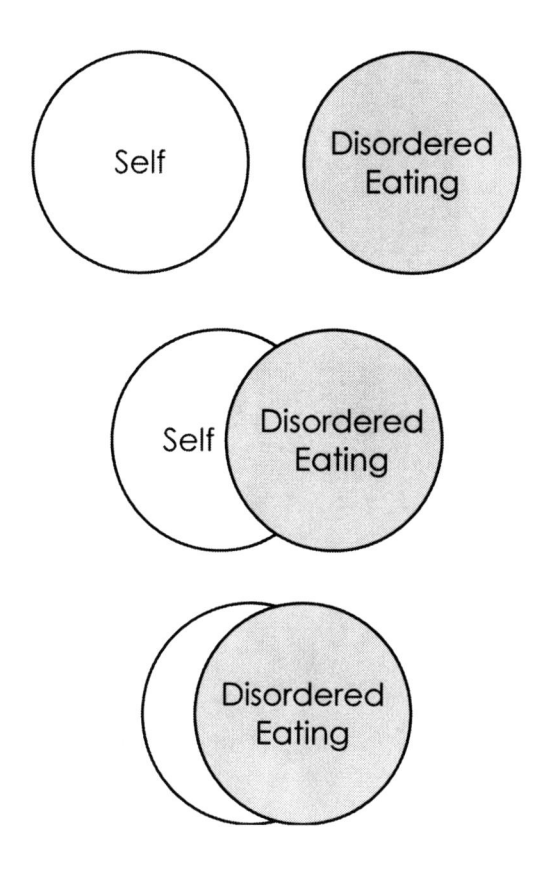

Externalisation gives you leverage against The Internal Terrorist. Having the problem appear to be separate makes it easier to defend yourself against any harsh internal criticism and allows more scope for possible solutions. It is easier to come at the problem from a different perspective. It is easier to challenge any negative thoughts and be less judgmental about any actions. Here is a sample from one of my client's externalisation exercises:

| Internal Dialogue (From the Internal Terrorist) | A Thought Challenge (From the Kinder, Gentler Self) |
| --- | --- |
| - I am fat.<br>- I am a disgusting pig.<br><br>- My thighs are too big. | - I am lovely.<br>- I am a beautiful and unique human being, there is no one like me anywhere.<br>- I may not like my thighs right now, but I can choose to accept them. Acceptance is neutral and will help me heal. |

Principle Five: Motivating Yourself for Change

**Happetite Training**

Exercise Thirty-Three:

Create your own Venn Diagram. Use one of these three options:

1. Draw your own Venn Diagram on a piece of paper. Draw a circle to identify you as the self and another circle in a different colour describing how much of your life gets taken up by disordered eating behaviours.

2. The Venn Diagram Worksheet Maker:

http://www.teach-nology.com/web_tools/graphic_org/venn_diagrams

3. You can also take counsellor and dietitian, Tara MacGregor's creative approach to this and make a 3-D version of it by taking a piece of cardboard, cutting a slit down the middle, and attaching circles that represent "the self" and "the problem". With the use of a simple peg, the circles slide over one another giving you some perspective on how the problem is eating up your life. Pun intended. See Appendix 5 for a template and directions.

Exercise Thirty-Four:

This exercise is about understanding the Internal Terrorist's dialogue and then deciding if you would like to defend yourself against it. There are four parts to this exercise.

1. In the left hand column in the chart on the next page write down the adjectives, words and phrases your Internal Terrorist uses.

2. In the right hand column write your thought challenges. Ask yourself: How might I challenge this Internal Terrorist? What kind of a debate can I have with the Internal Terrorist? What words would be more helpful or even the opposite of what I have written? Continue to add to these columns as you become aware of your internal dialogue. If you have a particularly strong Internal Terrorist you may need someone to help you with this exercise.

3. Take note of the themes and narrow them down to a few key words from the right hand column e.g. I am beautiful or I always nourish myself.

4. When you think you are in a place to start challenging your negative thoughts, try this: Eyeball yourself in the mirror and say the key, kind words to yourself. No protests that you don't believe it, beliefs are things we make up. This experiment is about trying something new. Pretend your way into a new reality. We perform to the level of our own self image and you are trying out a new self image around food, weight and shape. Experiment with using these as your daily mantras.

| Internal Dialogue (From the Internal Terrorist) | A Thought Challenge (From the Kinder, Gentler Self) |
|---|---|
| | |

Principle Five: Motivating Yourself for Change

## *Happetite Hints: Principle Five*

Prochaska's five stages of change include pre-contemplation, contemplation, preparation, action and consolidation.

There is an ebb and flow between the stages of change. Accepting where you are at in the stages of change is a key principle in making changes to your life around food, eating, weight and shape.

Four themes crucial in engaging in recovery include psycho-education, examining the advantages and disadvantages of the symptoms, the use of experimental strategies, and exploration of personal values.

Being free of food, weight and shape concerns means taking responsibility for your life, your eating and your response to physical, psychological, and mental triggers.

Externalising helps with the process of observation and making change.

# *Principle Six: Reconnect With Your (Perfect) Weight*

*"Rather than continuing this pointless effort to either fight our biology or stifle the free market, the best way to get over our weight problem is to stop worrying so much about our weight."*
-J. Eric Oliver in Fat Politics: The Real Story Behind America's Obesity Epidemic

## Lesson 20: Weighty Issues: Determining Your Perfect Weight

Let me define perfect weight. It is the weight your body wants to weigh. If that is hard to hear, ask yourself this: what if someone suggested that you lose five or ten centimetres off your height? What would you say to them? If someone asked you to buy a pair of shoes that were two sizes too small, what would you say to them about that? Vicki Hewson, the counselor and social worker I work with at Total Health Care often asks this question: "What would you do if someone asked you to change your eye colour?" If you have blue eyes and someone told you they needed to be brown or vice versa, what would you say? Expecting your body to be anything other than its natural weight is just as unrealistic.

Is it possible the current obsession with dieting and weight is a Westernised version of footbinding? If you have any doubt that restrictive dieting has similarities to footbinding read the amended version of the quote below from Beverly Jackson's Splendid Slippers. As a practice, footbinding began in the 10th Century AD in the Southern Tang Dynasty of China. It was first used among the elite and only in the wealthiest parts of China. It survived for nearly a thousand years until a small group of women in the late 1850s started to protest against it. And it was finally banned in 1911 after more than of one thousand years of being in vogue. I am hoping restrictive dieting doesn't stay in fashion that long.

---

**Similarities Between Chinese Footbinding and Restrictive Dieting?**

"For well over a thousand years, Chinese men and women pursued the ideal known as san zun jin lian, the three-inch golden lily, or golden lotus, as it is also called. The driving force behind this desire was complex: it had to do with marriage; it had to do with sex; it had to do with status; it had to do with beauty; it had to do with duty. Whatever the rationale, the fact is that by the time the practice was abandoned, millions of Chinese women had endured the unimaginable pain of the footbinding process, and in doing so, had sacrificed forever their ability to move about freely and normally." [From *Splendid Slippers* by Beverly Jackson, p. 24]

*My amended version:*

For well over a century, western men and women pursued the ideal known as thinness. The driving force behind this desire was complex: It had to do with marriage; it had to do with sex, it had to do with status, it had to do with beauty, it had to do with health, it had to do with duty. Whatever the rationale, the fact is that by the time the practice was abandoned, millions of Western men and women had endured the unimaginable pain of the dieting process, and in doing so had sacrificed much pleasure, inner peace and freedom.

## Principle Six: Reconnect With Your (Perfect) Weight

Our weight is genetically determined almost as specifically as our height or our shoe size. All three are variable.
- Our height shifts from morning to evening and over a lifetime.
- Our shoe size shifts from morning to evening. We are advised to buy shoes late in the day to accommodate for these changes in size.
- Our weight, when it is within our natural range, will fluctuate a couple kilograms up and down, even within the course of a day.

I remember discovering that people from The Netherlands are among the tallest, genetically, on the planet. I was visiting some friends in Amersfoot, Holland and as we wandered down one of the pedestrian streets I realised I was looking *up* at nearly everyone. I am quite tall and was not used to that. I had another sort of experience when I visited Spain and spent some time clothes shopping. I could not find a single piece of clothing that fitted me. *Everything* was too small and nearly everyone was much shorter. What examples do you have from your own life that supports this idea that some things come down to genetics?

**Commentary on Weighty Issues: Determining Your Perfect Weight**
In this section we are going to start exploring what your perfect weight might be. Please hang in there with me through this section. If I had to pick one area of recovery that offers up the most challenge for clients, I would say it is the notion of letting go of a desired, hoped for, or "fantasy" weight.

This area is a minefield of controversy and for many clients it is the most difficult hurdle. Thinking you need to be a certain weight will prevent you from recognising natural cues for hunger and satiety. You will be weighing yourself and worrying about your weight rather than accessing your natural hunger and satiety cues. Your body is very smart if you listen to it.

Major influences on weight and shape are your:
- Genetics
- Height
- Bone structure
- Metabolic rate
- Food habits
- Activity levels and
- Natural weight.

Your natural or perfect weight is the weight you will tend to be when you are eating in a basically healthy way and by that I mean listening to your body cues, eating a wide variety of food and taking care of yourself physically (i.e. being active on a regular basis). It varies from person to person and naturally increases with age until early adulthood. As an adult it will tend to stabilise at a level that may vary a few kilograms from month to month but if you are eating to your appetite it will be fairly steady over your life. Hormonal changes during menopause also affect women's weight, so it is important to manage the symptoms of menopause. Hormonal changes during pregnancy, lactation and the post-pregnancy period also trigger mood and food issues that can affect your weight. Take action early if you notice any abnormal weight changes or significant mood changes during these times.

How do you determine what your perfect weight might be, especially if you have been dieting or concerned with weight and shape for much of your life? What if you have never experienced your normal weight? Here are a few things to consider when determining what your natural weight might be:

1. A normal, healthy weight is a *range* and not one weight.
2. Medical and statistical analysis may be used as a *starting point*.
3. Adequate levels of sex hormones are required.
4. Nutritional needs vary from person to person.
5. Physical activity is meant to be fun – not a requirement.

## Principle Six: Reconnect With Your (Perfect) Weight

Let's explore each of these in a little more detail.

**1. A normal, healthy weight is a *range* and not one weight.**

When working with clients I usually discuss the idea of an initial target with them. If someone is underweight we may set a target range of BMI 20 + 2 Kilograms. While this may seem unrealistic if someone is very underweight and terrified of eating it is also a 'voice of reason' against the Internal Terrorist. Most people will not be able to eat to their appetite until they are well nourished.

If someone is overweight I suggest setting a target of slowing weight gain and perhaps halting it, before setting a weight target. Because of the cycle of hormone disruption that occurs once you are overweight, expecting weight loss while normalising eating habits is somewhat unrealistic. Of course, before either of these can be tackled, the wish for weight loss must be challenged (see Lesson 5). Hope can be held for long term success by focusing on the underlying causes, encouraging more normalised eating and activity, and looking for ways to increase metabolic activity.

**2. Medical and statistical analysis may be used as a *starting point*.**

- Body Mass Index for adults
- Growth charts for children and adolescents
- DEXA (Dual Xray Absorbtiometry) scans for more in-depth information

Body mass index equals weight in kilograms over height in metres squared (for Americans weight in pounds minus 703 over height in inches squared).

$$BMI = \frac{Weight\ (kg)}{(Height\ (m)^2)}$$

For example if someone weighs 69 kilograms and is 169 centimetres tall:

$$\frac{69 \text{kg}}{(1.69 \text{ m} \times 1.69 \text{ m})} = \frac{69 \text{ kg}}{2.85 \text{ m}} = \text{BMI of } 24.2 \text{ kg/m}^2$$

or

$$\text{BMI} = \frac{\text{Weight (lb)} - 703}{(\text{Height (in)}^2)}$$

There are also several internet sites that allow you to calculate your BMI easily. One that uses both Imperial and Metric formulas is The (U.S.) National Heart Lung and Blood Institute. (http://www.nhlbisupport.com/bmi/)

A BMI of 20-25 (19-24 for those with Asian backgrounds) is considered a good starting point; however in order for some people to be able to eat to their appetite their weight may fall outside of the normal BMI range. If that describes you, it is important to accept that your natural weight may not be in the 'normal' range. In our culture it seems easy to accept a weight that is *below* the reference range BMI of 20-25, but very challenging to be above it. The distinction here is if you are eating to your appetite your weight is likely to be close to or within the healthy weight range.

For those under 18 years, height and weight percentile growth charts may also be used to assess a healthy weight range. BMI increases naturally during adolescence. It can be assessed with a BMI for age chart.

A DEXA scan (Dual Energy X-ray Absorptiometry) can refer to either a regional study of the bone density of the hips and spine or can be a whole body scan that assesses total body bone mineral density and highly accurate measures of the body's soft tissue composition - muscle mass and fat mass. The whole body scan can provide extra information to help your medical team determine what your healthy weight might be.

## Principle Six: Reconnect With Your (Perfect) Weight

**3.** Adequate levels of sex hormones in adolescents and adults are required for normal body functioning.

If you have lost too much weight your body may stop producing male and female sex hormones. Women who are underweight may lose their menstrual flow. When you regain weight, normal hormone levels return and menstrual flow returns.

If you are carrying weight above your natural weight, your body may be releasing excess levels of hormones and perpetuate a cycle of further weight gain followed by further release of hormones.

**4.** Nutritional needs vary widely from person to person.

Are you able to eat enough nutritious food to get you through each day with plenty of energy? Are you getting a variety of foods to keep you healthy? If you are eating regularly and sufficiently you will be less preoccupied with food and weight concerns. Meeting the nutritional needs for ongoing growth (for children and adolescents) and maintenance (for adults) is important.

**5.** Participation in physical activity - if you are physically able - for the joy of it, without being compulsive about it.

Children are naturally active and never equate exercise with food or weight. They run around for the sheer joy of it. What would life be like if you could tap into that way of being again?

If you are preoccupied or compulsive about activity then it is likely that your weight is too low. High levels of activity can lower body fat to an unhealthy level where hormone levels will be affected. If you have grown sedentary over the years because increasing weight has made it more difficult to move your body, then your challenge is to find ways to safely and progressively engage in joyful movement like walking, swimming, aqua aerobics, dancing or perhaps some activity you used to engage in as a kid. As mentioned previously, Felicity Spencer, the physiotherapist at the Meridian Clinic, recommends yoga, tai chi and Pilates.

Numbers, numbers, numbers.

Weight in kilograms, pounds, stones? Sizes in France, America or Brazil? Energy in Kilojoules or Kilocalories?. In matters of weight, shape and food, if the numbers matter, then you are most likely out of touch with what your body needs and wants. If you desire a weight that is outside the limits of what your body wants to weigh or if you are obsessed with the fat content of the foods you are eating you may need a reality check. Numbers will not matter once you start listening to your intuitive body signals.

## Principle Six: Reconnect With Your (Perfect) Weight

**Happetite Training**

Experiment Thirty-Five: Letting Go of the Scale

Achieving detachment about your weight will help you reconnect with your appetite. If you are used to weighing yourself regularly, what would it be like for you not to know your weight? Set up an experiment where you gradually decrease the number of times you weigh yourself. You might also consider using the "Yay! Scale" – a scale that substitutes words like beautiful, perfect, gorgeous, adorable and sexy instead of numbers. Everyone who stands on it smiles. How cool is that? It is available from Voluptuart - a company that sells art and gifts that inspires you to celebrate your body. (www.voluptuart.com)

If on the other hand, you avoid weighing yourself out of fear, how might you allow yourself to be weighed and not let it determine the kind of day you have? If this experiment is too difficult to do on your own, seek the help of a skilled dietitian or therapist.

Exercise Thirty-Six:

Using the chart on page 203 identify ages and weights and identify what your highest and lowest weight has been. If you are an adult your natural weight will most likely be somewhere between these two numbers. The exceptions are people with persistent eating disorders that started in childhood, including obesity. If that describes you then some expert help will be required to help you determine what your natural weight might be. If you are under 18, using the National Center for Health Statistics (NCHS) growth chart will be much more helpful. When used appropriately, growth charts are a very valuable tool. However there is potential for misuse and misinterpretation. For that reason, even though you can download the charts, I strongly recommend you speak with your family doctor or dietitian so they can help interpret the charts correctly. The currently used charts have been scientifically developed based on a North American population by the NCHS, in Maryland, USA. You can download updated versions from the Centers for

Disease Control website: www.cdc.gov/growthcharts. Children from Asia tend to be smaller than North American children. As a result, a child of Asian background may seem to always be below average when plotted on these charts.

## Principle Six: Reconnect With Your (Perfect) Weight

| Age | Weight | Note highest and lowest |
|-----|--------|-------------------------|
|     |        |                         |
|     |        |                         |
|     |        |                         |
|     |        |                         |
|     |        |                         |
|     |        |                         |
|     |        |                         |
|     |        |                         |
|     |        |                         |
|     |        |                         |
|     |        |                         |
|     |        |                         |
|     |        |                         |
|     |        |                         |
|     |        |                         |
|     |        |                         |
|     |        |                         |

## Lesson 21: Media Mayhem

*"Why not be oneself? That is the whole secret of a successful appearance. If one is a greyhound why try to look like a Pekinese?"*
-Dame Edith Sitwell

### Commentary on Media Mayhem

By now we are all aware of the way the media re-touches photographs and creates unrealistic expectations. The Dove Real Beauty Campaign has done a brilliant job in showing the public what happens when products are marketed to them. But we buy into it anyway. We buy the products touted by beautiful people and we buy magazines with the slimmest women on the cover.

Cyndi Tebbel was the Editor of the Australian edition of *New Woman* magazine until she put a size 16 woman on the cover and lost advertising dollars.

Here's what she says:

"In the past few years, a couple of brave models have spoken out about the pressures of working in the fashion industry. Yet the business of fashion continues to invalidate the natural physiological evolution for members of the female gender. The way Mother Nature planned it, most of us start out life as slender girls and grow (repeat: grow) into wiser, wider and wrinkled women. But the pressure faced by models – to stay young, thin and beautiful forever – now affects all women regardless of age or profession". -from *The Body Snatchers*

Here are some American statistics that may prompt you to be more accepting of your weight: The average American woman is 5'4"(162.5 cm) tall and weighs 140 pounds (63.5 kg); the average American model is 5'11" (180 cm) tall and weighs 117pounds (53 kg). Most fashion models are thinner than 98% of American women. Four out of five American women say they are dissatisfied with the way they look and nearly half the women in the United States are on a diet on any given day.

Other scary statistics: almost half of American children between the first and third grade say they want to be thinner. Four

## Principle Six: Reconnect With Your (Perfect) Weight

out of five 10-year olds are afraid of being fat. On any given day one in four men are on a diet. The number of people living with eating disorders and disordered eating is triple the number of people living with AIDS.

There are some interesting positive changes afoot, at least in Australia. Perth magazine Silver uses no retouching. A recent Marie Claire magazine, with former Miss Universe Jennifer Hawkins on the cover in all her nude glory, created a media storm when it was announced the photo was not retouched. And for the first time at the fashion shows in Melbourne and Sydney in 2009 there were size 12-16 women modeling clothes on a couple of the catwalks. While certainly still the exception, it is great to see that the envelope of conformity is being stretched.

### Lesson 22: Letting Go of Expectations

> *"We cannot change anything unless we accept it.*
> *Condemnation does not liberate, it oppresses."*
> *-Carl Gustav Jung*

I have a difficult question to pose now. How can you accept your body, especially when it may not fit the cultural ideal? What if, due to your physiology, your weight will never fit the cultural ideal? Here is where things can get a bit sticky.

### Commentary on Letting Go of Expectations

My younger brother John has a wry, dry sense of humour. He overuses, in a very funny way, one of his favourite adages: "The secret to life is not having expectations". This from a man who has set and achieved many life goals.

The secret to life and recovery from food, weight and shape concerns is not having expectations about your weight. Your weight will take care of itself if you are taking responsibility for the other aspects.

Acceptance of your current weight is important. Acceptance has a much different tone to it than resignation or denial. Resignation has a sense of complacency attached to it, an acquiescence to one's fate. Denial is associated with disowning. Acceptance provides possibility. Acceptance provides space for self-care and positive feelings to arise.

Here is advice from one of my clients, N.B., as she neared the end of recovery:

"The initial motive to stop bingeing was to get thinner – but that won't ever work. What works is letting go of the need to lose weight, focus on the mind aspect, stopping the disturbed thoughts, and allowing normal eating. That's what eventually helped me break the cycle of bingeing."

## Happetite Training

<u>Exercise Thirty-Seven:</u>
Check out the Health at Every Size (HAES) information available on the internet. (www.haescommunity.org)

For women, explore the information available from the range of books published by Trinny and Susannah. Trinny Woodhall and Susannah Constantine are two British fashion advisors and bestselling authors who give advice and provide guidelines on improving appearance through the way you dress. They suggest styles that flatter each person's unique shape.

## *Happetite Hints: Principle Six*

Your perfect weight is the weight your body wants to be.

There are many similarities between the current practice of restrictive dieting and the ancient Chinese practice of footbinding.

Our natural weight is genetically determined like our height and eye colour. Other influences include food habits, activity levels and hormonal changes.

If you have never experienced your normal weight there are a few things to consider:
   A normal, healthy weight is a range and not one weight.
   Medical and statistical analysis may be used as a starting point.
   Adequate levels of sex hormones are required.
   Nutritional needs vary from person to person.
   Physical activity is meant to be fun, not a requirement.

The media impacts the social and cultural ideal we carry with us.

Letting go of expectations about changes to weight is important. Focus instead on the behaviours required to eat naturally and re-engage your happetite.

# *Principle Seven:*
# *Finding Your Happetite*

*"The difference between ignoring my appetite and eating to my appetite is the difference between being dead and being alive."*
-P.T., Client

Here is where we start putting everything together. By the end of this chapter you will have a set of clearly defined goals to move away from disordered eating and into the realm of Happetite.

**Lesson 23: Revisiting the Eating Continuum**
Your task in this lesson is accepting where you are on the Eating Continuum and deciding where you want to go.

**Commentary on Revisiting the Eating Continuum:**
Later on in the chapter you will be exploring in detail how to incorporate guidelines or a meal plan into your life. While treatment using guidelines and/or a meal plan is not normal eating, the aim is to help you replicate the structure inherent in appetite-driven eating. In turn that will help you re-establish a healthy relationship with food and eating.

The first step is acknowledging where you are and taking responsibility for that. Back in Exercise One on page 46, I asked you to mark where you thought you were on the continuum. Have you noticed any changes since then? Have your food rules intensified or lessened? Where are you on the continuum today? Mark it on the continuum below. Can you 'radically accept' where you are at? If so, great – move on to the next lesson. If not, then you will need to explore your motivation for change. Please review Principles Four and Five. See if you can move to a place of acceptance. Perhaps you need some support in doing that. Who might be able to help you?

Without adequate motivation the next steps will be daunting. Please continue to work on your motivation for change before moving further.

| Anorexia Nervosa | Restricted Dieting | Restrained Eating | **Guidelines or Meal Plan** | Normal Eating | Conscious Eating | Normal Eating | **Guidelines or Meal Plan** | Over-eating | Binge eating | Bulimia Nervosa |
|---|---|---|---|---|---|---|---|---|---|---|
| | | | | | ***Appetite Driven Eating*** | | | | | |
| External References (Food Rules) ||| | Internal References (No Food Rules) ||| | External References (Food Rules) |||

## Lesson 24: Using Your Normal Eating Style As a Template For Your Happetite Plan

All of us have eaten normally according to internal references of appetite at one time even if it was only the first few weeks of life before our environment interfered. It is your body's preference and automatic response to eat to appetite.

Everyone has a different definition of normal eating so how do you find what is normal for you as an individual? Every culture, every family, every individual has grown up with a set of principles and practices that guide their food choices and eating behaviours. How do you figure out what is right for you? How do you find *your* happetite? Your goal in this lesson is to find out what your eating and food choices might look like if your appetite was fully operational.

## Commentary: Using Your Normal Eating Style As a Template For Your Happetite Plan

In Lesson 3 you filled out a form called Your Dieting History on page 66. Look back at that now. Is there anything in your dieting history that did not trigger the starvation syndrome or the diet-binge cycle? Were there any specific aspects that you think you might want to take with you into your life with happetite? For example some techniques like chewing well and setting your fork down between bites are sometimes used to focus attention inwards. What might work for you now?

Write your ideas here:

_____

_____

_____

_____

Back in Lesson 8, on pages 103-105, I asked you to write down several different eating patterns you may have experienced:
- Your current eating;
- Your most restrictive or excessive eating; and
- Your normal eating (prior to any food, weight or shape concerns) if you had experienced that.

Complete them now if you have not already done so. If you have not ever eaten normally, or can't remember if you have, you can move on to the next lesson.

Compare what your eating is like now compared to when you ate normally. Do you eat less or more now than you did when you ate normally, or does it depend on the day? Was there structure in your normal eating? Typically, normal eaters will be eating regularly throughout the day, but some just munch along with no set pattern.

Note your answers here:

_____

_____

_____

_____

_____

_____

## Lesson 25: What's Your Plan: Structural or Observational?

The whole premise of Find Your Happetite is based on the wisdom of your body and the need to challenge any food and weight rules you have lived with. Because so many fears surface as you start to challenge your beliefs, some structure can be very helpful. But that structure is not normal eating, it is only a means to an end. There is a dialectic* needed here, an ability to hold two differing points of view at the same time. In this instance the dialectic is:

'Nutrition is everything and nutrition is nothing'.

---

* Dialectical Behaviour Therapy (DBT) was devised by Marsha M Linehan, a psychology researcher at the University of Washington. DBT seeks to find a balance between acceptance and change strategies in therapy and forms the fundamental "dialectic" – dialectic being a form of argument having its origins in ancient Greece.

## Commentary on What's Your Plan: Structural or Observational?

There are two main ways to gain access to your natural appetite:

1. Using observation.

2. Using some structure.

Some people may prefer to start recovery by tracking what is happening through the use of food/mood/appetite records and making adjustments towards normal eating based on what they find. Some may prefer general guidelines, and others may find that structuring a meal plan will be the most helpful starting point. How and when you decide to use the different modalities depends on your personality, your environment and the stage you are at in treatment.

First I'll address the benefits of simple observation and then look at the way some structure might work.

## Using Observation

**With observation the aim is to record your food intake, thoughts, emotions and appetite levels and notice how they interact and impact one another.** Use one of the record keeping forms in Appendix 2.

Observation itself can prompt change; that is why food/mood/appetite records are so beneficial for some people. Simply by objectively observing how your patterns of eating relate to your internal and external references you may notice a path to recovery. How you keep and use the record is important. Aim to record a full day or two at a time so you can start to identify habits and patterns. Take it easy - do not force yourself to do it. Stay curious. Be objective. Be non-critical. Be honest with yourself. Remember to use the positive parts of your self. Get help with interpreting the information if you need to.

## Using Structure

**With structure the aim is to set up a daily intake that will drive normal appetite signals out of hiding and let you get familiar with them while still having a 'safety net' to fall back on when the disordered eating presents itself.**

To set up the structure I usually suggest three nets, each with a finer weave:
Net One:    Structure of your environment.
Net Two:    Structure for the day.
Net Three: Structure for each meal and snack.

### Net One –The Structure of Your Environment

Here are some suggestions for creating a supportive environment for recovery:
- Surround yourself with support.
- Eat in a relaxed setting.
- Create a positive atmosphere at mealtimes.
- Eat with your family or friends at regular mealtimes if possible.
- Weigh yourself in a way that is consistent with the stage you are in treatment- that means you may not want to have scales in your home.
- If you are prone to overeating or binge eating you may want to eat those "fear foods" in a safe environment at first - perhaps with a friend or family member. Buying some foods in single serving portion sizes may also be helpful.

### Net Two - The Structure For the Day

There are two principle ways of setting up the structure of the day - either general guidelines or a more specific meal plan.

#### Using General Guidelines

The idea behind use of the general guidelines is that knowing a few nutrition basics and having a bit of structure will make learning to eat to your appetite a little easier.

- Aim to eat THREE meals plus THREE snacks about THREE hours apart. For most people appetite will work in two to three hour cycles, that is: if you eat to a modest level of satisfaction you will be hungry again in two to three hours so "Thinking Three " seems to help.
- Eat some protein, carbohydrate and fat at each meal. Use the lists on pages 220-224.
- Eat some carbohydrate and whatever else takes your fancy at snacks.
- If you avoid, feel deprived of, or fear certain foods you need to include these avoided or feared foods regularly. This is "exposure therapy" and the only way to eliminate the fear or feelings of deprivation. See Exercise 15, page 91.

**Using a Meal Plan**

The structure of a meal plan is something to experiment with – it is never rigid and aims for flexibility within the structure. Like an earthquake-proof building it remains structurally sound even if there are upsets or challenges. The aim of the structure is to reacquaint you with your appetite and help you stay out of the emotional cycle of guilt and deprivation. The meal plan will ideally be set up to move you from your current eating pattern back to your normal pattern of appetite-driven eating.

**Net Three – The Structure For Each Meal and Snack:**

Getting some protein, carbohydrate and fat at each of the main meals and enough nourishment at snack times to sustain you until the next meal is very helpful in re-establishing a connection to your natural appetite. Regular intake of protein, fat and carbohydrate helps get your metabolism and appetite working. Plant foods are given special status because of their nutrients and enzymes, but there are no rules. If you are craving pickles or chocolate for breakfast go for it. And then notice, as objectively as possible, what happens to your appetite throughout the day. The next lesson will look in detail at how these 'macronutrients' work together to help you get in touch with your internal references for hunger and satiety.

**In Practice**
  **Claire**

Claire was a 20-year-old in recovery from Anorexia Nervosa. She was still struggling to come to terms with much of her childhood abuse and would cycle between restrictive phases and binge eating phases. Eventually she got to a stage where she had gained enough weight that her appetite became apparent and she started to trust a meal plan as binge prevention. She began experimenting with eating normally but she had a constant overwhelming craving for chocolate. Though it was one of the foods she had denied herself for a long time, her craving for it was greater than any of the other foods she had avoided. Eventually, even though she was eating to her meal plan most days, she continued to binge on chocolate. In fact, it was about the only thing she was bingeing on. Try as hard as she might to feel okay about eating chocolate she continued to feel out of control around it. She could not let go of the guilt if she did eat it and deprivation if she didn't. She had tried to include chocolate as a part of her regular intake, first in the evening and then for her afternoon snack as well, but still ended up bingeing on it. So at one of our sessions we set up a meal plan of chocolate. Three meals and three snacks a day of chocolate. ('Blasphemy', I can hear you say.) She chose her favourite chocolates in the amounts that she thought would satisfy her. A week later she came back saying that after three days she was able to go back to her usual meal pattern because she'd had her fill of chocolate. She had not binged on chocolate all week. She needed to feel that she could eat whatever she wanted and the structure of the meal plan gave her some safety in experimenting with that. Cravings always send us signals that a physical, emotional or mental need is not getting met. What are your cravings telling you?

## Happetite Training

<u>Experiment Thirty-Eight:</u>
Set up your three safety nets:
Net One:   Structure of your environment.
Net Two:   Structure for the day.
Net Three: Structure for each meal and snack.

What do you need in your environment to make it safe to re-engage with your happetite? Experiment with the guidelines, a meal plan or food/mood/appetite records as a way of setting up structure through the day. Notice how the structure of meals will determine how hungry or satisfied you are throughout the day.

<u>Experiment Thirty-Nine:</u>
If you wish to experiment with a meal plan use your normal eating pattern which you wrote out on page 105 as a guide or use a pattern of three meals and three snacks spaced two to three hours apart. A session or two with a dietitian who uses a non-dieting approach may be very helpful in carrying out this experiment.

## Lesson 26: Nutrition Basics: Guidelines for Engaging Appetite

*"Nutrition is bound to life, to health and hope, to growth and healing, to hunger and suffering, to joy and vigour but always to being alive."*
-Lenor Morrett Surenos

## Commentary on Nutrition Basics: Guidelines for Engaging Appetite

When you have been out of sync with your appetite for many months or years it can be challenging and confusing having to start nourishing yourself again. But sound appetite regulation depends on your ability to nourish yourself and provide your body with adequate fuel.

Protein, carbohydrate and fat are the three main nutrients in food. They are called macronutrients because we need them in large amounts, and each has a different role to play in keeping us healthy, satisfied and listening to our appetite

These three macronutrients provide satiety – the feeling of satisfaction after eating. They provide satiety in different ways and at different times after a meal. Sugar is quickly absorbed, leaving the stomach quickly and provides satiety in the 20-30 minutes after a meal. Some of the more complex carbohydrates, now often termed low glycaemic index foods, have a slower uptake. Protein foods are slower still. Fat is the last of the nutrients to be digested and absorbed. Once it reaches the small intestine, fat stimulates the release of cholecystokinin, a hormone that signals satiety.

Studies on the glycaemic index of specific foods and meals (of satiety, viscosity and other measures of food uptake) give us *information* about how our bodies use the food we eat, but information alone won't give us an experience that helps us trust our own signals of hunger and satiety. The *experience* of hunger and satiety and the ability to respond to those signals is what helps change our relationship with food. Our beliefs and concerns around food, eating, weight and shape will change when we have new *experiences*. This is why the experimental approach is so crucial in finding your happetite.

The point of experimenting with regular meals and snacks is to help you get used to your normal appetite signals. How long does it take to learn to listen to your appetite? It depends on your situation; some people let go of their fears quickly and easily slide into eating according to their appetite. For others it can take months or even years. It takes courage, so be gentle with yourself. How long it takes is how long it takes.

Let's have a closer look at the macronutrients:

**Protein**

Amino acids are the component parts or building blocks of proteins.

Proteins provide the building blocks for your body.
Proteins are the brickwork in the factory that is your body.
Proteins are used for growing and repairing cells.
Proteins are needed to make:
- Enzymes, which help us digest food properly;
- Hormones, which help us to use stored energy;
- A strong immune system, helping us to fight infection and
- Cellular structure.

*Every* single cell is built with protein.

Not eating enough protein can be devastating to the body. We lose muscle as the body breaks down existing cells in order to create the raw materials it needs to function. Protein is important for satiety, those all-important feelings of fullness. Protein can help us feel satisfied for longer periods of time.

Sources of protein include:
- Fish
- Chicken
- Turkey
- Beef
- Lamb
- Pork
- Eggs
- Dairy foods: milk, cheese, yogurt

Principle Seven: Finding Your Happetite

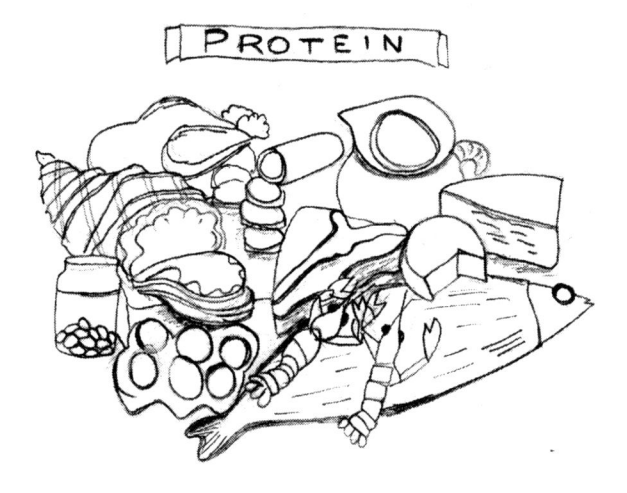

- Tofu
- Soy milk
- Nuts
- Legumes (lentils and other dried beans and dried peas)

**Carbohydrates**

These are your fuel for life. You happily fill the petrol tank in the car without guilt. If you set out on a long journey by car you make sure the engine is tuned and the petrol tank is full. What makes it so difficult to do the same with your body's own internal fuel gauge?

Carbohydrates are the main source of ready to go fuel. If you do not eat enough carbohydrate foods, blood sugar levels drop too low causing side effects including low energy levels, light headedness, loss of concentration, blurred vision and irritability.

Food cravings can develop, as can increased hunger, if you are not eating enough carbohydrate foods. Whatever the source of the carbohydrate, all break down into simple sugars including glucose.

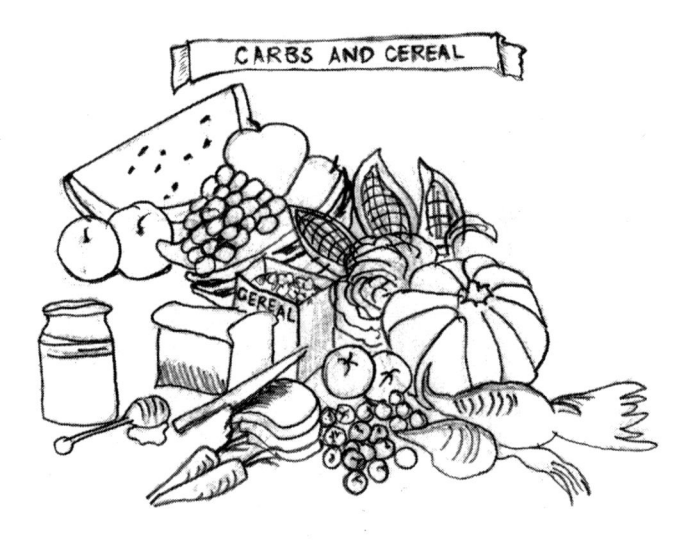

Sources of carbohydrate include:
- Breads
- Cereals
- Grain foods such as
  - Rice
  - Corn
  - Barley
  - Couscous
  - Pasta
  - Quinoa
- Vegetables* such as
  - Potato
  - Sweet potato
- Dairy foods
- Fruits
- Honey, syrup and other natural sweeteners and sugars

Many carbohydrate rich foods such as whole grain breads, cereals and potato are also significant sources of fibre. Fibre helps

---

* Other vegetables contain small amounts of carbohydrates but should not be the only carbohydrate included in a meal as they will not provide sufficient energy

keep our digestive tracts healthy and functioning well, prevents constipation and carries toxins from our body.

**Fat**

Fat is really very important, not the bad thing that our western world has come to believe. Fat, including oil, is the misunderstood kid waiting patiently for recognition. Fats in food provide essential fatty acids required for:
- Making hormones;
- Healthy skin;
- Brain cells (60-80% of the brain is composed of fat in the form of phospholipid sheaths);
- Carrying fat-soluble vitamins into the body and
- Adding flavor and texture to food.

The creamy feel of many foods is due to the fat in them. Not eating enough fat can trigger overeating. Fats cause the release of the hormone cholecystokinin (CCK). CCK is responsible for triggering satiety; it tells you when to stop eating. This is an important factor in normalising eating.

In the absence of adequate dietary fat - and protein - the body is forced to obtain vital nutrients and energy by breaking down muscle. A very low fat diet will often leave you feeling hungrier. Like protein, fat helps slow down the rate at which your stomach empties thus leaving you satisfied longer.

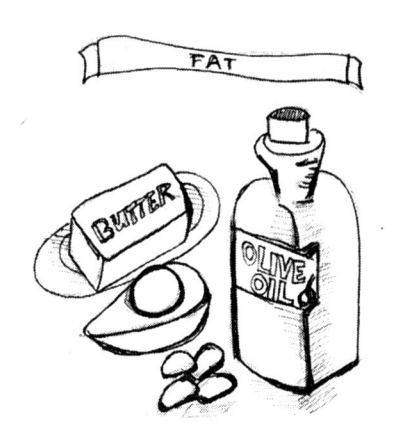

Sources of fat include:
- Oil
- Butter
- Margarine
- Avocados
- Fats in milk and dairy foods
- Fats in meats
- Fats in nuts, seeds and other proteins

Dieting, overeating and perhaps some over-used taste receptors from eating too many processed foods throw our internal mechanisms for hunger and satiety off balance. As mentioned before, all of our brain neurons are covered in a fatty sheath. This sheath is important for many reasons including appetite signalling. Ensuring you challenge any fears you have about eating fats will help you move towards your happetite.

## Principle Seven: Finding Your Happetite

**Happetite Training**

Experiment Forty:

Over four days compare how long you feel satisfied after the following four meals*. With each meal try to have the same overall amount of food. For example: eat one and a half cups of fruit on the first day, eat a total quantity of one and a half cups of fruit and nonfat yogurt on the second day, etc.
1. Day one: Fruit only. (carbohydrate)
2. Day two: Fruit with nonfat yogurt (carbohydrate and protein).
3. Day three: Fruit with regular yogurt. (carbohydrate, protein and fat)
4. Day four: Fruit with muesli and regular yogurt. (carbohydrate plus low GI carbohydrate, protein and fat)

Experiment Forty-One:

Interview someone you know who is a normal eater, someone who eats to their appetite and has no food, weight or shape concerns. This might be someone under school age! Find out what they know about the calorie content and nutritive value of foods. Usually only dieters, nutritionists and a few freakish biochemistry nerds will know these things. Find out how natural eaters make their decisions to eat or stop eating. Continue asking questions until you get some clues to the mystery of normal eating.

Experiment Forty-Two:

Using the food frequency chart on page 227 observe your eating for a couple of days. See how your meals stack up. What you are aiming for is a wide variety at each meal and through each day and week. As always, just observe. No judgment. If you notice some judgment or obsessive calculations creeping

---

* If you don't like fruit, yoghurt and muesli, experiment with foods you do like, making sure you get the nutrients in the order they are listed each day.

in discontinue the experiment. If it is helpful to you, there is a row at the bottom to do tallies at the end of the day. The wider the variety the happier your cells and body will be.

*"Let food be thy medicine and let thy medicine be food"*
*-Hippocrates*

## Principle Seven: Finding Your Happetite

| Protein foods | Carbohydrates | Fats | Vegetables | Fruit | Other Foods |
|---|---|---|---|---|---|
| Fish | Breads | Oil | Artichoke | Apricot | Add your |
| Chicken | Cereals | Butter | Bean | Apple | own list of |
| Turkey | Grain foods | Margarine | Beetroot | Banana | Preferences |
| Beef | such as | Avocado | Broad bean | Berry | here: (I'll |
| Lamb | -Rice | Fats in | Broccoli | Blackberry | get you |
| Pork | -Corn | milk and | Cabbage | Blueberry | started) |
| Eggs | -Barley | dairy | Carrot | Cherry | Ice cream |
| Milk | -Couscous | foods | Cauliflower | Cranberry | Cake |
| Cheese | -Pasta | Fats in | Celery | Currant | Chocolate |
| Yogurt | Potato | meats | Corn | Grape | Biscuits |
| Tofu | Sweet potato | Fats in | Cucumber | Grapefruit | Lollies |
| Soy milk | Dairy foods | nuts, seeds | Eggplant | Gooseberry | Bakery/ |
| Nuts | Fruits | Others: | Garlic | Lemon | Patisserie |
| Legumes | Honey | | Kale | Mandarine | items |
| Others: | Syrup | | Kohlrabi | Melon | |
| | Sugars | | Lettuce | Orange | |
| | Others: | | Onion | Pear | |
| | | | Parsnip | Peach | |
| | | | Parsley | Pineapple | |
| | | | Pea | Plum | |
| | | | Pumpkin | Raspberry | |
| | | | Radish | Strawberry | |
| | | | Shallot | Sweet cherry | |
| | | | Small radish | Watermelon | |
| | | | Spinach | Wild strawberry | |
| | | | Swede turnip | Others: | |
| | | | Tomato | | |
| | | | Turnip | | |
| | | | Others: | | |

Exercise Forty-Three:
Deciding what to eat when you are recovering from food and weight issues can be a challenge. Planning ahead and having some standard choices from which to choose when it is time to eat can be helpful. When planning your menus, think about what you would choose if you hadn't ever had any food and weight concerns. Aim to include some protein, carbohydrate and fat at each of the main meals.

1. Plan and write out seven breakfast menus.
2. Plan and write out seven lunch menus.
3. Plan and write out twelve evening meal menus.
4. Plan and write out ten snacks.

Exercise Forty-Four:
It is very helpful to have some basic cooking skills in order to move towards more conscious eating. If you don't already know how to cook, get someone to teach you a few basics. Don't be afraid to ask someone - most good cooks love to share their knowledge. Or consider taking a cooking course.

**Lesson 27: Making Friends With Your Happetite**
Sarah stands at the refrigerator. The light spills out around her like a B-grade movie. The digital clock on the counter ticks over to 2:15. She woke from a dream, felt anxious and is now polishing off the remains of dinner. She numbly moves fork to mouth and quells the jumble in her chest. She has difficulty falling back to sleep later, feeling full and uncomfortable. The next morning she is tired and groggy as she gets the kids ready for school and makes her way to work at the hospital. 'How am I going to make ends meet?' she worried to herself.

Andrea steps on the scales at the weight club meeting. She slumps with disappointment when the numbers say 68.2 - she has gained half a kilo. There is a voice inside her head, angry at the injustice. All the sacrifices: working out at the gym, no snacks between meals and passing on wine at dinner. Now this slap in the face. The lady who is doing the weighing gives her a sympathetic look. Andrea would like to yell at her with rage, but she holds her tongue.

Pete walks through the front door and hangs the bag with his dance gear on the hook next to the door, hangs the keys on the smaller hook next to it. The dance instructor told him today he needed to lose just a bit more to be in contention. "Some strength would help, too!" he had called after him as he left the studio. Pete lays his hand on his flat stomach and acknowledges he is starving. He is a bit dizzy as he leans over to pull the stainless steel pots from the drawer. He runs water into the bottom pot and sets it on the stove to boil. Steamed vegetables and a small rubbery piece of chicken leftover from the night before would be his dinner. He would get the part even if he had to do sit-ups all week.

Sarah, Andrea and Pete are all within their healthy weight range. They do not purge, they try to take care of themselves, and they all have disordered eating. They are managing their lives with food. They are managing their thoughts and emotions with food. They are not listening and responding to their bodies. Their cues for food come from outside themselves. They are unable to move away from thinking about food, weight and shape for much of the day. Each has a way of eating, none that are appetite driven. Typical dieting fits into the disordered eating end of the spectrum. You feel guilt if do eat, deprivation if you don't. If eating is entirely linked to listening and responding to the appetite and goes beyond normal appetite-driven eating to include healthy, conscious-choice decisions about food then it will not trigger either the starvation syndrome or the diet-binge cycle so common amongst dieters. This is the path we would all like to be on.

**Commentary on Making Friends with your Happetite**

As you learn to re-engage with your appetite there will be fears that arise out of the Internal Terrorist part of you. Fears such as:

"Even if I do get normal signals for hunger and satisfaction I will not be able to respond to them – I know I will overeat."

"I will never be able to trust my body."
"I can't trust my appetite."
"I feel anxious if I'm too hungry or too full."
"I will lose control of my eating and weight."
"I will become fat if I listen to my appetite."

Now is the time to move through your fear and into a place of power. Now is the time to experiment with the ideas and exercises in this section and learn to re-engage with your appetite. Now is the time to begin trusting your body again.

The first step is being able to recognise hunger and satisfaction signals. For some a simple Likert Scale is helpful:

1--------2--------3--------4--------5--------6--------7--------8--------9-------10

Nothing   Running      Hungry        Satisfied     Full     Overly
Left      Out                                               Full

For others the use of more descriptive words and phrases is helpful:
- I'm feeling faint: I've waited too long.
- I'm a little dizzy, fuzzy vision: I need something NOW.
- Not thinking clearly, lagging energy: I'd better eat because I'm hungry.
- I could eat a little more.
- I've eaten to my heart's content.
- No hunger left now, I'm full.
- I've overeaten and I can't eat another bite.
- I've really overdone it. I need to lie down.

Still others prefer to think of their appetite as a fuel gauge. The gauge tells you when to refuel. When the gauge reads full, you would not add more. When the gauge reads half-full, you may add some fuel but there is not any urgency to do so. When the gauge reads empty, you fill up. Are there other ways that you can think of to gauge your hunger and satisfaction levels throughout the day?

## Principle Seven: Finding Your Happetite

What do you do when the gauge is broken? Do you take precautions and perhaps carry fuel with you? Or for peace of mind do you repair the gauge? When it comes to re-engaging with your appetite, I encourage you to do both. (Technically you won't be repairing your appetite, only removing any obstacles that prevent you from listening to it.) Start carrying some food with you so you can readily respond to your emerging hunger signals.

How hungry are you right now? Take a moment to answer. Trust yourself, even if in your mind, the Internal Terrorist is telling you not to. If you have ignored your appetite for some time, it may take a little while to identify your level of hunger or fullness. Perhaps close your eyes so you can focus on the physical sensations. If you did not have food or weight concerns how hungry would you be? For most people it will help to take a little time to centre yourself before and after a meal. Ask yourself, "How hungry am I?" For people who are significantly underweight, weight recovery is necessary before appetite signals will work properly.

When working normally, appetite is a fairly sub-conscious mechanism. Just like the fuel gauge in the car, you don't really take notice of how helpful it is until it isn't working. For a relatively short time, if all goes well and you can get out of your mind's way, you will have to ask yourself this question consciously. This is why recording appetite levels before and after meals is very helpful for some people. It helps you stay focused and checking on your internal fuel gauge.

For some reading hunger is easy, understanding when to stop eating is more challenging. Do you have difficulty identifying when you are satisfied? Do you eat quickly and find that you overeat because satisfaction signals need time to register? Do you know when you are full, but keep eating anyway because there is food on the plate? A few recent studies suggest people with a certain gene (FTO) are more likely to override satiety cues when food is present. That means it is easier for people with this genetic type to keep eating even when they are already full. For these people having some structure in their environment is important, for example removing leftovers from the table when you are finished eating. The structure of the meal plan can also be helpful. To complicate matters further, being underweight can trigger early satiety -feeling full before you actually are full. This is why it is helpful to work with someone you trust to challenge anything that keeps you stuck in your eating habits. In the long term, paying attention and responding to your appetite is the key to recovery. It is all about observing and then experimenting with new ways of being that are in alignment with what you want.

The long-term aim is to work towards eating when you are hungry and stop eating when you are satisfied. This allows you to maintain your weight. So rather than appetite and weight swinging like a heavily loaded pendulum from one side of the continuum to the other, your appetite and weight settle.

---

The complexities of appetite described:

Psychological, social and environmental factors, nutrients and metabolic processes and gastric contractions originate hunger signals. Eating, in turn, activates inhibitory signals to produce satiety. Because of the delay between the swallowing of food and the digestion of food, the satiety mechanism requires a short-term signal to prevent over-eating. This short-term satiety signal is activated by psychological factors (such as sensory-specific satiety), chemical senses (taste and smell) and mechanical factors related to the process of swallowing and gastric distension. The long-term satiety is then activated by the chemoreception of nutrients and peptides by the gastrointestinal system (including the liver), the CNS (Central Nervous System) and by intrinsic CNS mechanisms.

-Plata-Salaman C, *Regulation of Hunger and Satiety in Man.*

## Principle Seven: Finding Your Happetite

**In Practice**
**Emma**

Referred by a dietitian who was moving to another city, Emma had a 12-month history of Anorexia Nervosa. With expert guidance over the previous six months and much effort on Emma's part, she had managed to regain 10 kilograms. She was within a kilogram or two of her minimum weight range (BMI 20 +2 kg) on the day I first saw her. She reported high anxiety about both changing dietitians and learning how to eat to her appetite again. She was still eating to a meal plan and terrified of what would happen if she started listening to her appetite. Emma had a strong memory of how she ate before the eating problems. She had been a natural eater and had never had weight concerns previously. Our first few sessions focused on how to make the transition from the safety net of the meal plan back to normal appetite regulation.

The concept of a Likert Scale of hunger was introduced. The scale ranged from 1-10 with 1 = ravenous, 10 = stuffed full. Emma asked to take the handout home with her. However she didn't relate to the numbers on the sheet. In fact looking at the scale deepened her panic about eating to her appetite. She was kinesthetically oriented and the numbers didn't mean anything to her. Fortunately she had a strong relationship with a skilled therapist and at their session the next day they translated the numbers into physical sensations that Emma experienced – for example when she was ravenous she felt dizzy, when she was stuffed full she felt groggy. Instead of keeping food records, she started keeping a record of how she felt before and after meals. She was weighed at her weekly appointments and discovered that her weight did indeed stay within the range we had identified as being the range her body likely wanted to weigh. There was a small glitch one week when she was prescribed pain medications for a medical issue; the pain disappeared along with her ability to recognise her appetite signals. The pain medications altered the signals between her brain and her body. A few days after she stopped the pain medications her appetite returned to normal. Once she understood that her appetite could be trusted; she was able to let go of her food and weight rules for good.

## Happetite Training:

Experiment Forty-Five:
Use the hunger and satiety scale. Notice how you feel before and after meals. You may want to make a record of this to see if there are patterns. Even if you don't believe it at first, trust you are right about your perceptions. Keep taking note until you make a discovery.

Experiment Forty-Six:
Have you tested out Experiment Thirty-Five from Lesson 20: Letting Go of the Scale? If not, revisit that now. Achieving detachment about your weight is an important step in recovery. If you are always thinking and worrying about your weight, it will be harder to listen and respond to the signals your body is sending. Have the courage to stop weighing yourself. If your eating and weight concerns are still potent, a skilled dietitian is the perfect person to assist you in challenging fears about weight gain and you can be weighed during regular consultations.

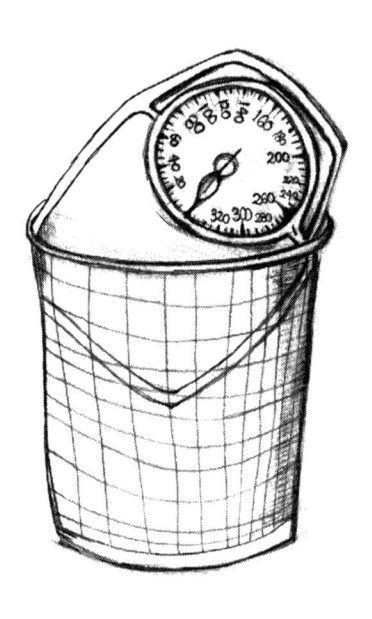

Exercise Forty-Seven: Visit Internet Websites That Support Recovery
Check out www.findyourhappetite.com, the Diet No More website: www.dietnomore.com.au or one of the other websites listed in Appendix 3 for other practical tips.

## Lesson 28: Move Your Body
How much do you move during the day? Physical activity patterns can fit into a continuum much like eating. Compulsive

activity is on one end and minimal or no activity on the other end of the scale. Somewhere in the middle is a pattern of activity that is natural and joyful and keeps the body in good health.

**Commentary on Move your Body**

What are your activity patterns like right now? Where are you on the continuum? If you didn't have weight concerns, what kinds of activity would you be doing?

| Compulsive exercise / Over-exercise / Rigid patterns | Naturally active / Consciously active / Naturally active | Mostly sedentary / Sedentary / No activity |
|---|---|---|
| External References (Exercise Rules) | *Joyful, Healthful Activity*<br><br>Internal References (No Rules) | External References (Exercise Rules) |

Research shows a distinct correlation between exercise and health (notice I said health, not weight). No matter what your weight, staying active can help keep you healthy.

> My little dog Louie does a 'downward dog' yoga position and a long body stretch along the spine every time he gets up from sleep. He also frequently, shakes off from head to toe. It seems remarkable to me that he stays standing, so violent is the shake. He does the shake after he relieves himself, after encountering other dogs, after being brushed. He shakes off after joyous situations and after difficult situations. Have you noticed how other animals and birds do this? I often wonder if we humans would be happier if we did a little more shaking.

Being active is especially important if you spend much time in front of the computer or on a mobile phone. When I visit my brother and his family in Wisconsin I hear my sister-in-law, Carol, advising my nephews to 'unplug' and go outside. Without movement, our bodies collect all sorts of energy - emotional, mental, physical - that has no where to go. Without movement, our mental, emotional and physical bodies become disrupted. An electromagnetic shift happens when we move our bodies. The yogis of India have known this for centuries. It has taken those of us in the West a little while to catch up. Because most of us cannot see energetic debris, it is hard to quantify it. We cannot see electricity, either; we quantify it by the output of energy. How often do you get out into nature to re-adjust the electromagnetic field of your body?

*"I have to admit I started yoga initially to lose weight, but through experience I've learned to let go of the ego and realise it's more emotional and spiritual in nature –the physical is a side benefit. It's helped me discover who I am and have a better picture of my life. After I practice I feel energized and I want to refuel my body in a healthy way."*
                                                            -A.R., client

## Principle Seven: Finding Your Happetite

**Happetite Training:**

Experiment Forty-Eight:

Make a list of all the physical activities you participated in and enjoyed before the advent of food, weight and shape concerns in your life. Remembering what you liked to do as a child can be helpful for some people.

Physical activities I enjoyed before I had food, weight and shape issues:

_____

_____

_____

_____

_____

Experiment Forty-Nine:

Consider where you are on the Activity Continuum. If you'd like to move to more conscious activity patterns what would you have to do? Could you perhaps set up an appointment with a physiotherapist or check out a yoga, pilates or tai chi class in your area? Write out any ideas you have below and then take one step towards your goal.

_____

_____

_____

_____

### Lesson 29: Moving Towards More Conscious Eating

Conscious-choice eating is very different from restrictive dieting. Your path never ends at the fork in the road that leads to either the starvation syndrome or the diet-binge cycle. When you are making food choices and eating from a place of conscious choice you have freedom around food, your eating is natural, you are not driven by guilt if you do eat, or deprivation if you do not eat. You have a harmonious relationship with yourself and your body.

Earlier in the book I described conscious-choice eating in the following way:

- ❏ Your eating is driven by appetite, the internal references of hunger and satiety and other internal cues.
- ❏ Your food choices are based on nutrition, the life force of food, and how food impacts your physical body and the planet.
- ❏ You make food choices intuitively, independent of other factors such as work schedule and social schedule.
- ❏ Your eating and food choices are in alignment with your core values and are self-nurturing.

How would you answer the questions of when, what, where, why and how would you eat? What would conscious-choice eating be like for you? Conscious-choice eating is based on your belief systems and values, therefore everyone will have a different answer to these questions.

### Commentary on Moving Towards More Conscious Eating

A few years ago I was lucky enough to travel with my documentary filmmaker friend, Maryella Hatfield, as she filmed a workshop on biomimicry. Biomimicry promotes the transfer of ideas inspired by nature to the design of our world, for a more sustainable, healthier planet. Janine Benyus coined the term and wrote the book *Biomimicry: Innovation Inspired By Nature* to describe the emerging field of bio-inspired innovation.

We met up with Janine and her training team deep in the throbbing jungle heart of the Amazon region in Peru at the

## Principle Seven: Finding Your Happetite

Tambopata Research Station. There we observed 24 designers from five continents using the Amazon rainforest to inspire solutions to their real design problems. The group included textile manufacturers from South Africa, architects from Syria and Boeing engineers from Seattle, amongst others. With no electricity, mobile phones, or wireless connections they used Nature as muse and model.

One of the many unexpected delights of that journey to Peru was the food. We were fed mouth-wateringly delicious foods with natural packaging. Never did we have to throw away any containers, plastic or paper. Grown locally, organically, and cooked fresh daily, it was full of life and nourishment.

We travelled by bus and boat for two days coming and two days going. We stayed for a week at the remote research station. For lunch one day on the boat, beautiful green parcels the size of a sandwich were passed out. Inside were slices of potato-filled omelet sandwiched with cheese and tomato. The omelet sandwich was wrapped in bijao leaves, large green pliable leaves much like a banana leaf. The green square was then tied up with a bit of dried vine, a beautiful gift of food with no waste. On the bus we were presented with a snack: A freshly picked orange and two perfectly roasted Brazil nuts in a locally made, re-usable covered basket. This description does little to evoke the experience of eating this vibrant, soul-satisfying food. At the research station homemade meals made from locally grown food were set out three times a day, fruit and freshly baked sweets for morning and afternoon snacks and a cup of tea before bed. Simple food cooked beautifully. Back in Sydney, I began thinking about how to move towards more sustainable, conscious eating. I began buying organic food whenever possible and always looked for foods with minimal packaging. I started asking myself how the food was going to impact my body and the planet.

How might Nature help you innovate and design a new way of being around food, weight and shape issues? How might you use Nature as muse and model to solve your concerns with appetite regulation?

I am inspired when I watch my little dog, Louie, eat. Every time I offer him something I am reminded how helpful nature is. He always takes his time. First he'll take a sniff, then a tentative taste. No matter how many times I've given him the food, he will first smell it. Then he will do one of three things: Step back and look at me as if to say, "Really? Isn't there anything better in the fridge?" or eat the food without much fanfare or heartily gobble it up.

## Happetite Training

<u>Exercise Fifty:</u>

Answer the following questions. If I ate with conscious-choice:

When would I eat?

_____

What would I eat?

_____

Where would I eat?

_____

Why would I eat?

_____

How would I eat?

_____

Now, in a sentence or two, summarise your ideas about what conscious-choice eating would be like for you:

_____

_____

_____

Note: your answers to these questions will change as you move through the layers of consciousness as described in the next chapter.

**List of Experiments and Exercises**
Tick off the list of exercises you have completed. Are there any you have avoided? What is your resistance to completing them? See if you can do what you resist. Doing what you resist will help you recover. Get support if you need it.

List of experiments and exercises (tick when completed):

- ❏ One: "X" on The Eating Continuum - the starting point to finding your happetite
- ❏ Two: "X" on The Eating continuum - other times in your life
- ❏ Three: If you have an eating disorder and not currently in treatment, seek help
- ❏ Four: Experimenting with acceptance
- ❏ Five: Practicing mindfulness
- ❏ Six: List of "shoulds" and "shouldn'ts" involving food
- ❏ Seven: Fill in The Diet/Binge Cycle Worksheet
- ❏ Eight: Fill in the Dieting History Worksheet
- ❏ Nine: Food, mood and appetite record keeping
- ❏ Ten: Observing how thoughts and feelings perpetuate the diet cycle
- ❏ Eleven: Clear out any diet foods, diet products and diet books
- ❏ Twelve: 'Dye-it' instead of diet the next time you want to lose weight
- ❏ Thirteen: Repeat exercise twelve every time you want to diet
- ❏ Fourteen: List your food, eating and weight rules
- ❏ Fifteen: List of food avoidances and challenging your food fears
- ❏ Sixteen: Writing out current and previous eating patterns

## Principle Seven: Finding Your Happetite

- ☐ Seventeen: Three-day record – physical effects of missed meals or overeating
- ☐ Eighteen: Documenting previous experiences of starvation or overeating after dieting
- ☐ Nineteen: Ticking physical consequences of starvation and overeating
- ☐ Twenty: Transit time test
- ☐ Twenty One: Experiment with solutions for constipation
- ☐ Twenty Two: Home thyroid test
- ☐ Twenty Three: Check-up with your doctor: TSH, BSLs and other concerns
- ☐ Twenty Four: If interested, have a hair tissue mineral analysis (HTMA)
- ☐ Twenty Five: Exploring normal eating
- ☐ Twenty Six: Additional information about your normal eating patterns
- ☐ Twenty Seven: Emotions related to eating normally
- ☐ Twenty Eight: Explore ways to begin releasing emotions
- ☐ Twenty Nine: Create your 'Joy List'
- ☐ Thirty: Start a 'Gratitude Journal'
- ☐ Thirty One: Motivational enhancement experiments
- ☐ Thirty Two: Filling in your honest appraisal worksheet
- ☐ Thirty Three: Create a Venn Diagram
- ☐ Thirty Four: Thought-challenging worksheet
- ☐ Thirty Five: Letting go of the scale
- ☐ Thirty Six: Weight history
- ☐ Thirty Seven: Explore Health at Every Size Information
- ☐ Thirty Eight: Set up three safety nets – structure of environment, day and meals
- ☐ Thirty Nine: Work out a meal plan using your normal eating pattern or work with a dietitian skilled in using a non-dieting approach
- ☐ Forty: Four-day satisfaction experiment – monitoring hunger and fullness
- ☐ Forty One: Interview a normal eater
- ☐ Forty Two: Food frequency chart
- ☐ Forty Three: Planning standard meal and snack choices

- ❏ Forty Four: Learn basic cooking skills
- ❏ Forty Five: Record appetite levels before and after meals and snacks
- ❏ Forty Six: Revisiting letting go of the scales
- ❏ Forty Seven: Visiting internet websites that support recovery
- ❏ Forty Eight: List of physical activities previously enjoyed
- ❏ Forty Nine: Your plan for conscious activity.
- ❏ Fifty: Your description of conscious-choice eating

## Principle Seven: Finding Your Happetite

### *Happetite Hints: Principle Seven*

**There are two main ways to gain access to your natural appetite:**
- Using observation; or
- Using some structure

With observation, the aim is to record your food intake, thoughts, emotions and appetite levels and notice how they interact and impact one another.

With structure, the aim is to set up a daily intake that will drive normal appetite signals out of hiding and let you get familiar with them while still having a 'safety net' to fall back on when the disordered eating presents itself.

**Knowing a few nutrition basics will make eating to your appetite a little easier:**

Aim to eat THREE meals plus THREE snacks about THREE hours apart. For most people, appetite will work in 2-3 hour cycles, that is: if you eat to a modest level of satisfaction you will be hungry again in 2-3 hours so "Thinking Three" seems to help.

Aim to eat some protein, carbohydrate and fat at each meal. Use the food lists.

Eat some carbohydrate and whatever else takes your fancy at snacks.

Aim to eat a wide variety of foods.

If you avoid, feel deprived of, or fear certain foods you need to include these avoided or feared foods regularly. This is "exposure therapy" and the only way to eliminate the fear or feelings of deprivation.

Observing and recording your appetite levels before and after meals with the use of a Likert Scale (or descriptive phrases) is a step towards learning how your body responds to food. It will help you build trust in yourself and your body.

Eating when you are hungry and stopping when you are satisfied is what allows you to maintain your weight.

Conscious activity is full of joy and is beneficial for you and your body. It is not compulsive and you do not feel guilt if you cannot exercise.

# *The Nature of Recovery*

*"Wake up, wake up, wake up"*
*-Yogi Bhajan*

Congratulations are in order! You have completed the seven principles and applied the lessons. You are well on your way to recovery. There are no lessons in this chapter, but personally, in terms of the work I do and the context I do it in, this chapter is fundamental. This may be the missing link to help you move off the dieting merry-go-round once and for all.

Though not a principle in and of itself, the spiritual nature of recovery from food, weight and shape issues is one of the more interesting parts of the process. Recovery from any form of disordered eating, including eating disorders, always involves transformation. Anyone who has lived with an eating problem or has lived with a child or teen who had an eating disorder, or food avoidance disorder, are forever changed by the experience. Once someone has come to terms with the food, eating, weight and shape issues that have plagued them, they are steadier and calmer in the face of other life difficulties.

Here in Australia, Year 12 students undergo what is called the "Higher School Certificate" (HSC), a series of exams that ultimately determine what college and career they can choose.

Typically most teens worry and panic over this series of tests, but one client who had recently recovered from an eating disorder had this to say:

> "All my friends were stressed, but I wasn't. Having the eating disorder was stressful, getting better was stressful. Everything else seems a walk in the park now."

Anyone who has been through a life-threatening illness and looked death in the face is changed. Many eating problems don't, on the surface, appear threatening to one's life, but they are. They block us off from listening to who we really are.

Ultimately finding your happetite is a spiritual journey because when you are intimately connecting, responding and trusting your happetite you are intimately connecting with the whole of your body, mind and soul. When you are intimately connected with these aspects of yourself in the physical realm (the physical, mental and emotional parts of your being) you are connected with who you really are. Who you really are is one aspect of the One, all-connected source energy, God, Yahweh, Jesus, or whatever divine nature sits best with your current experience.

No matter what your belief, it is our responsibility – our ability to respond - while we are in the physical realm, to be as connected to and honouring of our physical self as possible. As I was working on this chapter, I had a timely visit by two Fionas from Dublin. Fiona Horan, a friend of mine from her days living in Sydney and Fiona Fay, her business partner. Fiona Fay had just published a book: *Who is God? You Are*. The penny dropped for me about this link between acceptance and honouring of our physical, earthly nature and our higher, ethereal nature. The physical and non-physical always work in harmony.

> **An Irish Blessing**
> This beautiful blessing, handed down from the Middle Ages, is now used as a meditation to close Kundalini Yoga classes worldwide.
>
> *May the long time sun shine upon you,*
> *All love surround you,*
> *And the pure light within you,*
> *Guide your way on.*

## Here Are Some Possible Spiritual Blocks to Finding Your Happetite:

- ❏ Your "energy system" (etheric or non-physical body) may need balancing through yoga or some other physical or energetic work.
- ❏ Your physical symptoms have not resolved with allopathic medical care and healing from an alternative practice such as Reiki, homeopathy, acupuncture, Rekindled Ancient Wisdom (RAW: a form of energy balancing grounded in kinesiology), or one of the many other healing choices available on the planet may be helpful.
- ❏ Recognising the shadow. Look at what and who strongly repels or attracts us, we project both sides of the shadow onto those around us. Though psychological in nature, the shadow projection often has repercussions at a spiritual level.

## Levels of perception

Everything in the world has to do with energy and levels of perception. As humans we like to organise our world in ways that fit with our perception. Here are just a few theories, philosophies and ways of looking at the world. I am sure you can add to the list:

| Systems of Perception | Levels |
| --- | --- |
| Maslow's Hierarchy of Needs | 5 levels of human needs |
| Control Theory | 5 human needs |
| Vedic Science | 7 states of consciousness |
| Spiral Dynamics (Dr Clare Graves) | 8 levels + |
| Huna Philosophy | 7 principles |
| Chakra System | 7+ levels of being |
| Lynette Arkadie's Energy System | 10 layers of energy |

Each of these theories or systems is the result of a lifetime of research, experience and experimenting. Some like the Vedic scriptures are ancient; many are the result of intuitive 'knowing'. In fact many of the systems identified come from the non-physical realm and do not have time or dimension associated with them. The following brief summaries are in no way meant to reflect the complexity of any theory or philosophy, only a way of providing easy access to a few of the ways we humans organise our world.

## Maslow's Hierarchy of Human Needs (Motivational)

Abraham Maslow was an American psychologist whose main work throughout his life was identifying and defining a hierarchy of human needs. In order, they include:
- Physiological
- Safety
- Love and Belonging-Social
- Esteem
- Self-Actualisation

## Control Theory

Control Theory is a psychological theory arising from William Glasser's Reality Therapy. The five basic human needs according to control theory are:
- Survival
- Love
- Power
- Fun
- Freedom

## Vedic Science

Vedic science originated in Ancient India. The mystery of consciousness is explained and explored in the Vedas and Patanjali's Yoga Sutras. The seven states of consciousness as described by Vedic science are:
- Sleeping
- Dreaming
- Waking
- Transcendental
- Cosmic
- God
- Unity

**Spiral Dynamics**

This intriguing and complex organising system explains nearly everything in the universe. The eight systems originally described by Dr Clare Graves:

Survival, biogenic needs satisfaction, reproduction;
Safety/security, protection from harm, family bonds;
Power/action, asserting self to dominate others, control;
Stability/order, obedience to earn later reward, meaning;
Opportunity/success, competing to achieve results, influence;
Independence/self-worth, fitting a living system, knowing;
Harmony/love, joining together for mutual growth, awareness; and
Global community/life force, survival of Earth, consciousness;

**Huna Philosophy**

A philosophy that dates back to ancient Egypt, now most often associated with the Hawaiian kahunas (medicine men). The most fundamental idea in Huna philosophy is that we each create our own personal experience of reality, by our beliefs, interpretations, actions and reactions, thought and feelings. The seven principles are:

The world is what you think it is.
There are no limits.
Energy flows where attention goes.
Now is the moment of power.
To love is to be happy with.
All power comes from within.
Effectiveness is the measure of truth.

## The Chakra System

Chakra is a Sanskrit term meaning wheel. The chakra system is fundamental to traditional Indian medicine and yoga philosophy. Each of the major chakras is associated with a gland and major nerve plexus and governs the area of the physical body in which it is found. The Seven Major Chakras include:

- Base (tribal) chakra
- Sacral (creative and sexual) chakra
- Solar plexus (personal will and power) chakra
- Heart (love) chakra
- Throat (self expression) chakra
- Third eye (trust) chakra
- Crown (self essence and inspiration) chakra

## Lynette Arkadie's Energy System

Lynette Arcadie is a talented and natural spiritual healer. She and her business partner, Joy Moulieri, operate The Soul Factory and now run Energy Laundry Days in Sydney, Australia using a cycle Lynette devised by watching and understanding what helped and hindered her own and her client's energy fields. The ten levels/layers of energy are:

- Physical energies
- Mental energies – conscious, subconscious, unconscious
- Emotional energies
- Spiritual energies
- Soul energies
- Karmic and destiny energies
- Genetic and DNA level energies
- Core beliefs
- Past, present and future energies
- The communication system – how the systems relate internally and externally

What is your current perception of the world? Which systems appeal to you? Natali Jocelyn, a gifted Kundalini Dance teacher and therapeutic masseuse always tells me the way to the spiritual is through the physical. Taking care of and connecting with our physical self is one important aspect of "moving through the layers". This is why judgment never works. Any time we move out of acceptance of where we are, we are disconnecting from our higher self, the part of us that always knows how we might evolve and change. (This is where the dialectical approach is so helpful e.g. being able to hold both acceptance of where we are at and the possibility for change in equal measure.)

In the fable–like *Ringing Cedars of Russia* series, author Vladimir Megre recounts his story of meeting the Siberian recluse Anastasia, a descendent of the Vedrus (Russian Vedic line) and the subsequent life changing events triggered by his contact with her. Megre now speaks publicly about his experiences, encouraging others to move toward a more holistic approach to life. In his books he reveals how Anastasia's education on "divine nutrition" helped him recover from illness.

**Is Divine Nutrition Possible?**

Yes, I believe it is. It fits into the center of the eating continuum and is a step beyond conscious-choice eating. As human consciousness evolves and transcends the levels, so will the food we grow, harvest and eat. We will not be able to eat the foods we have been up until now, but will require a need for foods that fit with our newer higher vibration.

Bio-dynamic and other ways of growing things will help people understand the importance of the vibration or *life force* of the food, too (in scientific terms I believe this relates to the enzymatic properties found in food). Eating, and appetite, will become much more refined. We will make our food choices from a higher, divine place. We will be connected to the Infinite and make choices that fit with that level of perception.

For now, these are my hopes:
Every human will:
- ❖ Nourish themselves, and view themselves as worthy of nourishment.
- ❖ Eat to their heart's content.
- ❖ Feel contentment and satisfaction after eating.

- ❖ Live in peace with their physical body and speak lovingly when they look in the mirror.
- ❖ Farmers will provide reasonably priced unaltered organic foods. (Most food manufacturers will have to find something else to do, as food will be provided straight from the garden or the farmers nearby.)

In short, every human will:
Enjoy life, eat to their appetite and trust and love their body.

# *References/Sources*

Web site URLs are current as of December 2010.

**Introduction: The Seven Principles of Happetite**

Millions of people in the industrialised world spend billions each year on dieting:
> Though there are no figures from a reliable US government/research agency, a company called MarketData analyses the US weight loss market. They quote that 58.6 billion dollars was spent on the weight loss industry in 2009 and in 2010 it will be 68.7 billion. The company estimated the number of dieters (2009) was 72 million.

After dieting, most people regain most, if not all, their lost weight at 5 years:
> Anderson JW, Konz EC, Frederich RC, Wood CL. Long-term weight-loss maintenance: a meta-analysis of US studies. Am J Clin Nutr. 2001;74:579-84.

> Jeffery RW, Epstein LH, Wilson GT, Drewnowski A, Stunkard AJ, Wing RR, et al. Long-term maintenance of weight loss: Current status. Health Psychology. 2000;19:5-16.

More than 30% of the industrialised world's population is overweight or obese:

Flegal KM, Carroll MD, Ogden CL, Curtin LR. Prevalence and Trends in Obesity Among US Adults, 1999-2008. JAMA. 2010;303:235-41. (American adults (over age of 20) over BMI of 25 in 2008 was 68%, over BMI of 30 was 34%.)

Australian Bureau of Statistics. Overweight and Obesity in Adults, Australia. Canberra, ACT: Australian Bureau of Statistics, 2005. (54% of adults were classified as overweight or obese)

Up to one in five college women in the U.S. have an eating disorder: Between 11 and 20% of female American university students score high enough to indicate an eating disorder on the Eating Attitudes Test:

Nelson WL, Hughes HM, Katz B, Searight HR. Anorexic eating attitudes and behaviors of male and female college students. Adolescence. 1999;34:621-33. (20%)

Prouty AM, Protinsky HO, Canady D. College women: Eating behaviors and help-seeking preferences. Adolescence. 2002;37:353-63. (17%)

Thome J, L. Espelage D. Relations among exercise, coping, disordered eating, and psychological health among college students. Eating Behaviors. 2004;5:337-51. (11%)

Parts work:
Holmes, T. Holmes, L. Parts work: an illustrated guide to your inner life. Kalamazoo (MI): Winged Heart Press; 2007.

**Principle One: Understanding Your Eating**

Cycle Diagram adaptation
Coish, BJ. Anti-diet: you are not what you eat. Melbourne, Australia: Hill of Content. 1988; p 24-25.
(Quote Box)
Megre V. Anastasia (The Ringing Cedars, Book 1). Wetherall Park, Australia: Ringing Cedars Press LLC; 2008.

# References/Sources

Description of Acceptance and Commitment Therapy:
Harris, R. Embracing your demons: an overview of Acceptance and Commitment Therapy. *Psychotherapy in Australia* 2006; (Vol 12)4: 2-7

The passing on of maladaptive eating behaviours from parent to child:
Vogels N, Posthumus DLA, Mariman ECM, Bouwman F, Kester ADM, Rump P, et al. Determinants of overweight in a cohort of Dutch children. American Journal of Clinical Nutrition. 2006;84:717-24.

Birch LL, Davison KK. Family environmental factors influencing the developing behavioral controls of food intake and childhood overweight. Pediatr Clin North Am. 2001;48:893-907.

Fisher JO, Birch LL. Restricting access to foods and children's eating. Appetite. 1999;32:405-19.

Hood MY, Moore LL, Sundarajan-Ramamurti A, Singer M, Cupples LA, Ellison RC. Parental eating attitudes and the development of obesity in children. The Framingham Children's Study. Int J Obes Relat Metab Disord. 2000;24:1319-25

Whitaker RC, Deeks CM, Baughcum AE, Specker BL. The relationship of childhood adiposity to parent body mass index and eating behavior. Obes Res. 2000;8:234-40.

Dietary restraint as a maintenance factor in binge eating:
Bohon C, Stice E, Burton E. Maintenance factors for persistence of bulimic pathology: a prospective natural history study. International Journal of Eating Disorders. 2009;42:173-8.

"Feeling fat" leads to dietary restraint and subsequent eating disorders:
Cooper MJ, Deepak K, Grocutt E, Bailey E. The experience of 'feeling fat' in women with anorexia nervosa, dieting and non-dieting women: an exploratory study. European Eating Disorders Review. 2007;15:366-72.

Spear BA. Does Dieting Increase the Risk for Obesity and Eating Disorders? Journal of the American Dietetic Association. 2006;106:523-5.

Stein DM Reichart P Extreme dieting behaviours in early adolescence *J Early Adolescence* 1990; 10(20: 108-121

The negative emotions that come with "feeling fat":
Cooper MJ, Deepak K, Grocutt E, Bailey E. The experience of 'feeling fat' in women with anorexia nervosa, dieting and non-dieting women: an exploratory study. European Eating Disorders Review. 2007;15:366-72.

Most people with eating disorders diet before progressing to an eating disorder:
Striegel-Moore RH, Bulik CM. Risk Factors for Eating Disorders. American Psychologist. 2007;62:181-98.

People lose weight for mood or appearance reasons have lower psychosocial scores:
O'Brien K, Venn BJ, Perry T, Green TJ, Aitken W, Bradshaw A, et al. Reasons for wanting to lose weight: different strokes for different folks. Eating Behaviors. 2007;8:132-5.

People who lose weight for appearance reasons use more drastic measures and more dietary restraint:
Putterman E, Linden W. Appearance Versus Health: Does the Reason for Dieting Affect Dieting Behavior? Journal of Behavioral Medicine. 2004;27:185-204.

The importance of record keeping:
Shay LE, Shobert JL, Seibert D, Thomas LE. Adult weight management: translating research and guidelines into practice. Journal of the American Academy of Nurse Practitioners. 2009;21:197-206.

Shay L. Self-monitoring and weight management. Online Journal of Nursing Informatics. 2008;12:10p.

# References/Sources

**Principle Two: Understanding Your Happetite**

Ability for babies and children to regulate appetite:
> Fomon SJ, Filer LJJr, Thomas LN, Anderson TA, Nelson SE. Influence of formula concentration on caloric intake and growth of normal infants. Acta Paediatrica Scandanavica 1975 64:172-181.
>
> Birch LL, Fisher JA. Appetite and eating behavior in children. Pediatr Clin North Am. 1995;42:931-53.

The interaction of fat (both ingested and body fat levels) and how they help regulate appetite:
> Woods SC, D'Alessio DA. Central control of body weight and appetite. J Clin Endocrinol Metab. 2008;93:S37-50.
>
> Sharkey KA. From Fat to Full: Peripheral and Central Mechanisms Controlling Food Intake and Energy Balance: View from the Chair. Obesity. 2006;14:239S-41S.
>
> Little TJ, Horowitz M, Feinle-Bisset C. Modulation by high-fat diets of gastrointestinal function and hormones associated with the regulation of energy intake: implications for the pathophysiology of obesity. Am J Clin Nutr. 2007;86:531-41.

Description of normal eating by Ellyn Satter:
> Satter, E. What is normal eating? (Online). 2009 (cited 2010 Mar); Available from: URL: https://ellynsatter.com/showArticle.jsp?id=268&section=753

Eating Competence:
> Satter, E. Eating competence: nutrition education with the satter eating competence model J Nutr Educ Behav. 2007;39: S189-S194.

Vegetarianism:
> O'Connor M.A., Touyz S.W., Dunn S.M. & Beumont P.J.V. (1987) 'Vegetarianism in anorexia nervosa? A review of 116 consecutive cases.' Med.J.Aust. vol.147:540-542

Robinson-O'Brien R, Perry CL, Wall MM, Story M, Neumark-Sztainer, D. Adolescent and young adult vegetarianism: Better dietary intake and weight outcomes but increased risk of disordered eating behaviors. JADA. 2009;Vol. 109, Issue 4: 648-655

**Principle Three: Clearing the Physical Challenges**

The starvation syndrome:
Keys A. Biology of human starvation / by Ancel Keys, Josef Brozek, Austin Henschel (and others) of the Laboratory of Physiological Hygiene, School of Public Health, University of Minnesota, with forewords by J. C. Drummond (and others). Minneapolis : University of Minnesota Press 1950.

The challenges of making people gain weight:
Sims EAH, Horton ES. Endocrine and Metabolic Adaptation to Obesity and Starvation. Am J Clin Nutr. 1968;21:1455-70.

Adrenal insufficiency test:
Wilson J. Adrenal Fatigue: The 21st Century Stress Syndrome. Petaluma, CA: Smart Publications; 2001.

On gluten withdrawal in hypothyroidism:
Sategna-Guidetti C, Volta U, Ciacci C, Usai P, Carlino A, De Franceschi L, et al. Prevalence of thyroid disorders in untreated adult celiac disease patients and effect of gluten withdrawal: an Italian multicenter study. Am J Gastroenterol. 2001;96:751-7.

On high cholesterol and hypothyroidism:
Diekman T, Lansberg PJ, Kastelein JJ, Wiersinga WM. Prevalence and correction of hypothyroidism in a large cohort of patients referred for dyslipidemia. Arch Intern Med. 1995;155:1490-5.

Gut transit times:
Hasler WL. The Physiology of Gastric Motility and Gastric Emptying. In: Tadataka Y, editor. Textbook of Gastroenterology. 5th ed. ed. Hoboken, NJ: Blackwell Pub; 2009. p. 207-30.

Hasler WL. Motility of the Small Intestine and Colon. In: Tadataka Y, editor. Textbook of Gastroenterology. 5th ed. ed. Hoboken, NJ: Blackwell Pub; 2009. p. 231-63.

Low AG. Gut transit and carbohydrate uptake. Proc Nutr Soc. 1988;47:153-9.

Fructose malabsorption
   Shepherd SJ, Gibson PR. Fructose malabsorption and symptoms of irritable bowel syndrome: guidelines for effective dietary management. JADA 2006;166:1631-1639.

Hypothyroid test
   Barnes, BO. Hypothyroidism: The Unsuspecting Illness. Harper Collins; 1976.

Hair tissue mineral analysis:
   Tabrizian, I. Practitioners guide to reading a tissue mineral analysis. NRS Publications Series. Revised 2nd ed.

Xenoestrogens:
   Goldner WS, Sandler DP, Yu F, Hoppin JA, Kamel F, Levan TD. Pesticide use and thyroid disease among women in the Agricultural Health Study. Am J Epidemiol. 2010;171:455-64.

   Alavanja MCR, Sandler DP, Lynch CF, Knott C, Lubin JH, Tarone R, et al. Cancer incidence in the agricultural health study. Scand J Work Environ Health. 2005;31 Suppl 1:39-45; discussion 5-7.

   Chavarro JE, Toth TL, Sadio SM, Hauser R. Soy food and isoflavone intake in relation to semen quality parameters among men from an infertility clinic. Hum Reprod (serial on the Internet). 2008: Available from: http://humrep.oxfordjournals.org/cgi/content/abstract/den243v1.

**Principle Four: Addressing the Emotional Barriers**

Psychological symptoms from under-eating:
Keys A. Biology of human starvation / by Ancel Keys, Josef Brozek, Austin Henschel (and others) of the Laboratory of Physiological Hygiene, School of Public Health, University of Minnesota, with forewords by J. C. Drummond (and others). Minneapolis : University of Minnesota Press 1950.

Bruch: refeeding before doing other therapy:
Bruch H. Conceptual confusion in eating disorders. Journal of Nervous and Mental Disease. 1961;133:46-54.

Bruch H. Eating disorders : obesity, anorexia nervosa, and the person within. London (England): Routledge & Kegan Paul; 1974.

Emotional intelligence:
Hein S. Definition of Emotional Intelligence (Online). 2005 (cited 2010 May 27); Available from: URL:http://www.eqi.org/eidefs.htm

Bradberry T, Greaves J, Lencioni PM. Emotional Intelligence 2.0. San Francisco (CA): Publishers Group West ; 2009.

Meditation/transcendental meditation:
Wallace RK, Benson H. The physiology of meditation. Scientific American. 1972;226:84-90.

Benson H. The relaxation response / (by) Herbert Benson with Miriam Z. Klipper. Klipper MZ, editor. London: Collins; 1976.

Wallace RK, Dillbeck M, And EJ, Harrington B. The effects of the transcendental meditation and tm-sidhi program on the aging process. International Journal of Neuroscience. 1982;16:53-8.

Wenneberg SR, Schneider RH, Walton KG, Maclean CRK, Levitsky DK, Salerno JW, et al. A Controlled Study of the Effects of the Transcendental Meditation® Program on Cardiovascular Reactivity and Ambulatory Blood Pressure. International Journal of Neuroscience. 1997;89:15 - 28.

The sedona method:
: Dwoskin, H. The sedona method: your key to lasting happiness, success, peace and emotional well-being. Sedona (AZ): Sedona Press; 2003.

The joy list:
: Power AM. How To Stay Positive (Online). 2007 (cited 2010 May 27); Available from: URL:http://www.soulmentoring.com/positive.html.

Gratitude journal:
: Ban Breathnach S. Simple Abundance: a daybook of comfort and joy. New York (NY): Warner Books; 1995.

## Principle Five: Motivating Yourself for Change

Quote (Bose):
: Yogananda P. Autobiography of a Yogi. 11th ed. Los Angeles: Self-Realization Fellowship; 1972.

Body image in adolescence carries into adulthood:
: Zbornik S, Rockwell C. Sex differences and variations in Body Attitudes. Unpublished thesis. University of Wisconsin – Department of Educational Psychology; 1988.

  Slater A, Tiggemann M. The Contribution of Physical Activity and Media Use during Childhood and Adolescence to Adult Women's Body Image. J Health Psychol. 2006;11:553-65.

Body image is stable in adulthood:
: Tiggemann M. Body image across the adult life span: stability and change. Body Image. 2004;1:29-41.

People desire weight loss even though they are at a normal weight:
: Strauss RS. Self-reported weight status and dieting in a cross-sectional sample of young adolescents: National Health and Nutrition Examination Survey III.(Erratum appears in Arch Pediatr Adolesc Med 1999 Sep;153(9):945). Arch Pediatr Adolesc Med. 1999;153:741-7.

McElhone S, Kearney JM, Giachetti I, Zunft HJ, Martinez JA. Body image perception in relation to recent weight changes and strategies for weight loss in a nationally representative sample in the European Union. Public Health Nutr. 1999;2:143-51.

Ryan YM, Gibney MJ, Flynn MA. The pursuit of thinness: a study of Dublin schoolgirls aged 15 y. Int J Obes Relat Metab Disord. 1998;22:485-7.

Jackson M, Ball K, Crawford D. Beliefs about the causes of weight change in the Australian population. Int J Obes Relat Metab Disord. 2001;25:1512-6.

Motivational enhancement stages of change:
Prochaska JO, Norcross JC, DiClemente CC. Changing for good: A revolutionary six-stage program for overcoming bad habits and moving your life positively forward. New York: Avon; 1994.

Dean HY, Touyz SW, Rieger E, Thornton CE. Group motivational enhancement therapy as an adjunct to inpatient treatment for eating disorders: A preliminary study. European Eating Disorders Review. 2008;16:256-67.

Touyz S, Thornton C, Rieger E, George L, Beumont P. The incorporation of the stage of change model in the day hospital treatment of patients with anorexia nervosa. European Child & Adolescent Psychiatry. 2003;12:i65-i71.

Vitousek K, Watson S, Wilson GT. Enhancing motivation for change in treatment-resistant eating disorders. Clinical Psychology Review. 1998;18:391-420.

Firewalking:
Kurek Ashley Success International. Team building: firewalking (online). 2008 (cited 2010 Aug 1); Available from: URL:http://www.kurekashley.com/wa.asp?idWebPage=13073&idDetails=106

Firewalking (box):
: Adams, C. Can you walk on hot coals in bare feet and not get burned? The Straight Dope 14 June 1991 (retrieved 23 April 2010), http://www.straightdope.com/columns/read/644/can-you-walk-on-hot-coals-in-bare-feet-and-not-get-burned

Narrative therapy:
: Morgan A. What is narrative therapy? : an easy-to-read introduction. Adelaide: Dulwich Centre Publications; 2000.

Externalisation:
: Schaefer J, Rutledge T, editor. Life without Ed : how one woman declared independence from her eating disorder and how you can too. New York: McGraw-Hill; 2004.

Venn diagram:
: Venn Diagram Worksheet Maker (Online). 2010? (cited 2010 May 27); Available from: URL:http://www.teach-nology.com/web_tools/graphic_org/venn_diagrams/.

**Principle Six: Reconnecting With Your (Perfect) Weight**

Introductory quote:
: Oliver JE Fat politics: the real story behind America's obesity epidemic, p. 188

Chinese footbinding:
: Jackson B. Splendid slippers: a thousand years of an erotic tradition. Berkeley, Calif: Ten Speed Press; 1997.

Major influences on weight and shape:
: Cameron N, editor. Human growth and development. Sydney: Academic Press; 2002.

Media influences (quote):
: Tebbel C. The body snatchers: how the media shapes women. Sydney: Finch Publishing; 2000.

Calculating reference weights:
   World Health Organization. WHO child growth standards: length/height-for-age, weight-for-age, weight-for-length, weight-for-height and body mass index-for-age: methods and development. Geneva: World Health Organization; 2006.

   Dietitians Association of Australia. Best practice guidelines for treatment of overweight and obesity in adults. Deakin ACT: Dietitians Association of Australia; 2004.

   Wakefield A, Williams H. Practice recommendations for the nutritional management of anorexia nervosa in adults. Deakin ACT: Dietitians Association of Australia; 2009

Calculating BMI:
   National Heart Lung and Blood Institute. Calculate Your Body Mass Index (Online). (2010?) (cited 2010 Aug 1); Available from: URL: http://www.nhlbisupport.com/bmi/

DEXA scans:
   Laskey MA. Dual-energy X-ray absorptiometry and body composition. Nutrition. 1996;12:45-51.

Hormonal changes during pregnancy, lactation and menopause that affect weight:
   Lovejoy JC. The influence of sex hormones on obesity across the female life span. Journal of Women's Health. 1998;7:1247-56.

Hormone disruption associated with overweight:
   Klein S, Romijn JA. Obesity. In: Kronenberg H, Williams RH. editors. Williams textbook of endocrinology. 11th ed. Philadelphia: Saunders/Elsevier; 2008.

Yay! scale:
   VoluptuArt: Art & gifts for celebrating your body. Yay! Scales (online). 2010 (cited 2010 Aug 1); Available from: URL: http://voluptuart.com/other-goodies-yay-scales-c-7_22.html

Marie claire magazine with Jen Hawkins on the cover:
February 2010 of Marie Claire Australian edition Interview available at:
http://au.lifestyle.yahoo.com/marie-claire/article/-/6642179/interview-jennifer-hawkins/

US weight statistics:
Inch-Aweight: weight loss and fitness. The average american woman dieting & weight statistics. (online). 2010 (cited 2010 Aug 1); Available from: URL: http://www.inch-aweigh.com/dietstats.htm

**Principle Seven: Finding Your Happetite**

Eating with family and friends:
Neumark-Sztainer D, Wall M, Story M, Fulkerson JA. Are family meal patterns associated with disordered eating behaviors among adolescents? J Adolesc Health. 2004;35:350-9.

Appetite and the FTO gene:
Wardle J, Llewellyn C, Sanderson S, Plomin R. The FTO gene and measured food intake in children. Int J Obes. 2008;33:42-5.

Wardle J, Carnell S, Haworth CMA, Farooqi IS, O'Rahilly S, Plomin R. Obesity Associated Genetic Variation in FTO Is Associated with Diminished Satiety. J Clin Endocrinol Metab. 2008;93:3640-3.

Carnell S, Wardle J. Appetitive traits in children. New evidence for associations with weight and a common, obesity-associated genetic variant. Appetite. 2009;53:260-3.

The complexities of appetite (box):
Plata-Salaman CR. Regulation of hunger and satiety in man. Dig Dis. 1991;9(5):253-68.

Importance of food variety:
Freeland-Graves J, Nitzke S. Position of The American Dietetic Association: Total Diet Approach to Communicating Food And

Nutrition Information. Journal of the American Dietetic Association. 2002;102:100-8.

National Health & Medical Research Council. Dietary guidelines for Australian adults. 3rd ed. Canberra: NHMRC; 2003.

Food variety influences healthy eating behaviour:
Westenhoefer J. Establishing dietary habits during childhood for long-term weight control. Ann Nutr Metab. 2002;46:18-23.

Positive effects of eating regular frequent meals:
Koletzko B, Toschke AM. Meal Patterns and Frequencies: Do They Affect Body Weight in Children and Adolescents? Critical Reviews in Food Science and Nutrition. 2010;50:100 - 5.

Larson NI, Neumark-Sztainer D, Hannan PJ, Story M. Family Meals during Adolescence Are Associated with Higher Diet Quality and Healthful Meal Patterns during Young Adulthood. Journal of the American Dietetic Association. 2007;107:1502-10.

Nicklas TA, Baranowski T, Cullen KW, Berenson G. Eating Patterns, Dietary Quality and Obesity. J Am Coll Nutr. 2001;20:599-608.

Sjoberg A, Hallberg L, Hoglund D, Hulthen L. Meal pattern, food choice, nutrient intake and lifestyle factors in The Goteborg Adolescence Study. Eur J Clin Nutr. 2003;57:1569-78.

Health and activity: The health risks are similar between fit men no matter what their weight:
Wessel TR, Arant CB, Olson MB, Johnson BD, Reis SE, Sharaf BL, et al. Relationship of Physical Fitness vs Body Mass Index With Coronary Artery Disease and Cardiovascular Events in Women. JAMA. 2004;292:1179-87.

Blair SN, Church TS. The Fitness, Obesity, and Health Equation: Is Physical Activity the Common Denominator? JAMA. 2004;292:1232-4.

Biomimicry:
Benyus JM. Biomimicry : innovation inspired by nature. New York: Perennial; 2002.

**The Nature of Recovery**

Maslow's hierarchy of needs:
  Maslow AH. Toward a psychology of being 3rd ed. New York: J. Wiley & Sons; 1999.

Glasser and control theory:
  Glasser W. Control theory : a new explanation of how we control our lives. New York: Perennial Library; 1985.

Graves and spiral dynamics:
  Beck DE, Cowan CC. Spiral dynamics: mastering values, leadership, and change, Cornwall: Blackwell Publishing; 1996.

Vedic knowledge:
  Maharishi Mahesh Yogi. Science of being and art of living: transcendental meditation. New York: Meridian; 1995

  Russel, P. The tm technique. London: Elf Rock Publications; 2002.

  Patanjali. (Feuerstein, G. trans). The yoga-sutra of patañjali: a new translation and commentary. Inner Traditions; 1989.

Huna philosophy:
  King, S.K. Mastering your hidden self: A guide to the huna way. Wheaten Ill: Quest Books; 1985.

Chakra system:
  Judith, A. Eastern body, western mind: psychology and the chakra system as a path to the self. Berkeley: Celestial Arts; 1996

Rekindled ancient wisdom:
> Ancient Perceptions. Rekindled ancient wisdom (online). 2003 (cited 2010 Aug 1); Available from: URL: www.rekindledancientwisdom.com.au

Lynette arkadie:
> The Soul Factory (online). 2010 (cited 2010 Aug 1); Available from: URL: http://www.thesoulfactory.com.au/The_Soul_Factory.html

Divine nutrition:
> Megre V. Anastasia (The Ringing Cedars, Book 1). Wetherall Park Australia: Ringing Cedars Press LLC; 2008.

# *Appendix 1: DSM IV Criteria for Eating Disorders*

**DSM-IV-TR Criteria for Anorexia Nervosa:**
- Refusal to maintain body weight at or above a minimally normal weight for age and height (e.g. weight loss leading to maintenance of body weight less than 85% of that expected; or failure to make expected weight gain during period of growth, leading to body weight less than 85% of that expected).
- Intense fear of gaining weight or becoming fat, even though underweight.
- Disturbance in the way in which one's body weight or shape is experienced, undue influence of body weight or shape on self-evaluation, or denial of the seriousness of the current low body weight.
- In postmenarcheal females, amenorrhea, i.e., the absence of at least three consecutive menstrual cycles. (A woman is considered to have amenorrhea if her periods occur only following hormone, e.g., estrogen administration.)

Furthermore, the DSM-IV-TR specifies two subtypes:
- *Restricting Type:* during the current episode of anorexia nervosa, the person has not regularly engaged in binge-eating or purging behavior (that is, self-induced vomiting,

or the misuse of laxatives, diuretics, or enemas). Weight loss is accomplished primarily through dieting, fasting, or excessive exercise.
- *Binge-Eating Type or Purging Type:* during the current episode of anorexia nervosa, the person has regularly engaged in binge-eating OR purging behavior (self-induced vomiting, or the misuse of laxatives, diuretics, or enemas).

## The ICD-10 criteria are similar, but in addition, specifically mention

1. The ways that individuals might induce weight-loss or maintain low body weight (avoiding fattening foods, self-induced vomiting, self-induced purging, excessive exercise, excessive use of appetite suppressants or diuretics).
2. Certain physiological features, including *"widespread endocrine disorder involving hypothalamic-pituitary-gonadal axis is manifest in women as amenorrhoea and in men as loss of sexual interest and potency. There may also be elevated levels of growth hormones, raised cortisol levels, changes in the peripheral metabolism of thyroid hormone and abnormalities of insulin secretion"*.
3. If onset is before puberty, that development is delayed or arrested.

## DSM-IV-TR Criteria for Bulimia Nervosa:
- Recurrent episodes of binge eating. An episode of binge eating is characterized by both of the following:
- Eating, in a fixed period of time, an amount of food that is definitely larger than most people would eat under similar circumstances. Mainly eating binge foods.
- A lack of control over eating during the episode: a feeling that one cannot stop eating or control what or how much one is eating.
- Recurrent inappropriate compensatory behavior to prevent weight gain, such as: self-induced vomiting; misuse of laxatives, diuretics, or other medications; fasting; excessive exercise.

## Appendix 1: DSM IV Criteria for Eating Disorders

- Triggers include periods of stress, traumatic events, and self-evaluation of body shape and weight.
- These symptoms may occur after every meal on a daily basis or once every few months.
- The disturbance does not occur exclusively during episodes of anorexia nervosa.

There are two sub-types of bulimia nervosa:
- **Purging type** bulimics self-induce vomiting (usually by triggering the gag reflex or ingesting emetics such as syrup of ipecac) to rapidly remove food from the body before it can be digested, or use laxatives, diuretics, or enemas.
- **Non-purging type** bulimics (approximately 6%-8% of cases) exercise or fast excessively after a binge to offset the caloric intake after eating. Purging-type bulimics may also exercise or fast, but as a secondary form of weight control.

### DSM-IV Criteria for EDNOS:
The EDNOS category include disorders that do not meet the criteria for a specific eating disorder. Each one of the following disorders is an example:
- For females, all of the criteria for anorexia nervosa are met except that the individual has regular menses.
- All of the criteria for anorexia nervosa are met except that, despite substantial weight loss, the individual's current weight is in the normal range.
- All of the criteria for bulimia nervosa are met except that binge eating and inappropriate compensatory mechanisms occur at a frequency of less than twice a week or for a duration of less than 3 months.
- The regular use of inappropriate compensatory behavior by an individual of normal body weight after eating small amounts of food (eg; self-induced vomiting after the consumption of two cookies).
- Repeatedly chewing and spitting out, but not swallowing, large amounts of food.

- Binge eating disorder: recurrent episodes of binge eating in the absence of the regular use of inappropriate compensatory behaviors characteristic of bulimia nervosa.

*Reprinted with permission from the Diagnostic and Statistical Manual of Mental Disorders, Fourth Edition, Text Revision, (Copyright 2000). American Psychiatric Association*

*Appendix 2:
Monitoring Forms*

# Find Your Happetite

## Understanding Your Eating (Dieters)

Date: _____ Day: _____

| Time | Thoughts and Feelings Before Eating | Hunger | Food Eaten and Fluids | Fullness | Location | Thoughts or Feelings After Eating |
|------|--------------------------------------|--------|-----------------------|----------|----------|-----------------------------------|
|      |                                      |        |                       |          |          |                                   |
|      |                                      |        |                       |          |          |                                   |
|      |                                      |        |                       |          |          |                                   |

Connections made between food, mood and appetite:

# Appendix 2: Monitoring Forms

## Understanding Your Eating (Eating Disorders)

Date: _____  Day: _____

| Time | Thoughts and Feelings Before Eating | Hunger | Food Eaten and Fluids | Fullness | Location | Thoughts or Feelings After Eating | B | L | V | E |
|---|---|---|---|---|---|---|---|---|---|---|
|  |  |  |  |  |  |  |  |  |  |  |
|  |  |  |  |  |  |  |  |  |  |  |
|  |  |  |  |  |  |  |  |  |  |  |
|  |  |  |  |  |  |  |  |  |  |  |
|  |  |  |  |  |  |  |  |  |  |  |

**B** = Binge
**L** = Laxatives
**V** = Vomit
**E** = Exercise

Connections made between food, mood and appetite:

# *Appendix 3: Resources*

**Websites:**

www.findyourhappetite.com

www.tcme.org The Center for Mindful Eating
As a practice, Mindful Eating can bring us awareness of our own actions, thoughts, feelings and motivations, and insight into the roots of health and contentment. While the purpose of the Center for Mindful Eating is to help professionals and institutions, there is a downloadable handout outlining the principles of mindfulness and mindful eating.

www.dietnomore.com.au
Diet No More is an established non-diet approach to eating and weight management. Judith McFadden, a psychologist, and her daughter Jenny McFadden, developed a unique program called NECTAR (Natural eating Control Theory and Results).

www.ellynsatter.com
Ellyn Satter pioneered the concepts of the feeding relationship and eating competence. As a registered dietitian and social worker in the U.S., she has combined her expertise in nutrition and psychology

to pioneer the field of feeding dynamics. Her business, Ellyn Satter Associates provides resources for professionals and the public in the area of eating and feeding. She offers professional training, publishes training materials, teaching resources and books for parents and professionals.

www.ifnotdieting.com.au
Dr Rick Kausman is a medical doctor who is recognised as one of the Australian pioneers of the person-centred approach to healthy weight management. His book If Not Dieting, Then What? along with this website aims to help people achieve and maintain a healthy, comfortable weight without being deprived of food or losing quality of life; and to enjoy food without feeling guilty.

www.jeanhailes.org.au
This website is devoted to women's health issues including but not limited to PCOS (polycystic ovary syndrome). The focus is on translating the latest research findings into practical health and lifestyle approaches for women and their health professionals

www.mhfa.com.au
Mental health first aid guidelines for dealing with an eating disorder. Guidelines designed to help members of the public provide first aid to someone who is developing or experiencing an eating disorder. The role of the first aider is to assist the person until appropriate professional help is received. From the MHFA training and research program at the Orygen Youth Health Research Center, University of Melbourne.

www.conectphysiotherapy.com
Felicity Spencer is a Physiotherapist who works with our team at the Meridian Clinic at Total Health Care. She recommends mindful movement practices such as yoga and tai chi, not only for conditioning the physical body, but also as a way to become more at peace with your emotions.

# *Appendix 4:*
# *Getting Help If You Have an Eating Disorder*

**In Australia**
The Centre for Eating and Dieting Disorders
www.cedd.org.au

The Butterfly Foundation
Melbourne:
PO Box 453
Malvern VIC 3144
Phone: (03) 9822 5771   Fax: (03) 9822 5776
Sydney:
103 Alexander Street
Crows Nest NSW 2065
Phone: (02) 9412 4499   Fax: (02) 8090 8196
www.thebutterflyfoundation.org.au

**In the United States**
National Eating Disorders Association
603 Stewart Street, Suite 803
Seattle, WA 98101
Toll Free Information and Referral Helpline: (800) 931-2237
Email: info@nationaleatingdisorders.org
www.nationaleatingdisorders.org

**In the United Kingdom**
BEAT (Beat Eating Disorders)
Wensum House
103 Prince of Wales Road
Norwich NR1 1DW
Tel: 0845 634 1313
www.b-eat.co.uk
email: help@b-eat.co.uk

# *Appendix 5: Externalising Activity/Venn Diagram*

### **Making a 3D Venn diagram**

What you will need: 2 sheets of heavy duty cardboard – in different colours.

    Scissors or x-acto knife
    The templates on the next two pages
    Coloured paper and coloured markers or pictures
        from magazines and glue
    A paper fastener

Cut two circles from one of the pieces of cardboard.

On one circle create (draw or cut and paste using the coloured paper or pictures from magazines) an image representing 'the disordered eating' and on the other circle create an image representing 'who you really are' without the eating issues.

Trace the rectangular template onto the other piece of cardboard.

Align and paste the centre point of the circle with the image representing 'who you really are' at one end of the centre line you have just traced onto the cardboard.

Cut out the center line on the square template (through the circle that is pasted on top). The cut should end at the centre point of the circle pasted on top.

Using the paper fastener (or hole punch) punch a hole through the middle of the other circle representing 'the disordered eating'. Place the two ends of the paper fastener through the centre line slit on the rectangular cardboard and flatten the paper fastener ends to the back of the cardboard.

The circle representing the eating disorder will slide along the cut out "track" and cover the circle representing who you really are.

Play around with this. Ask your self questions like: How much of who I am gets covered up during the day when I'm stressed about eating, when I'm at a dinner party and thinking about my weight, when I'm with friends and concerned about what food choices to make, etc.

This tool can be used to help you externalise the eating issues and look for ways to think differently about them. This externalising activity can be used for *any* problem and is particularly useful with children.

# Appendix 5: Externalising Activity/Venn Diagram

Circle template for Venn Diagram

CPSIA information can be obtained at www.ICGtesting.com
Printed in the USA
BVOW012224060512

289301BV00003B/1/P